Bundles of Joy

LINDA FAIRLEY

Bundles of Joy

Two Thousand Miracles.
One Unstoppable
Manchester Midwife.

This book is a work of non-fiction based on the author's experiences.
In order to protect privacy, names, identifying characteristics,
dialogue and details have been changed or reconstructed.

HarperElement
An imprint of HarperCollins*Publishers*
77–85 Fulham Palace Road,
Hammersmith, London W6 8JB

www.harpercollins.co.uk

and HarperElement are trademarks of
HarperCollins*Publishers* Ltd

Published by HarperElement 2012

1 3 5 7 9 10 8 6 4 2

A catalogue record for this book is
available from the British Library

ISBN 978-0-00-745714-4

Printed and bound in Great Britain by
Clays Ltd, St Ives plc

Find out more about HarperCollins and the environment at
www.harpercollins.co.uk/green

For Peter,
who told me I could do this.
He would be very proud.

Contents

'Go, and do thou likewise.'

Prologue

'She's on the bathroom floor!' Sarah's husband puffed as he flung open the front door and ushered me inside the house. 'Come in,' he said urgently, giving me a grateful smile. 'You must be frozen.' Turning his head towards the stairs, he shouted up to his wife, 'The midwife's here! Love, the midwife's here!'

Robin Heywood then turned on his heel and charged upstairs. I hastily pulled off my Wellington boots and winter coat and followed him, dripping water all over the carpet as I did so.

It was just before Christmas 2002 and I'd driven and trudged through deep snow to get here. Sarah Heywood hadn't planned a home birth and when her waters broke her husband had called an ambulance in the hope they could make it to Tameside Hospital, where she was booked in to have her baby.

Snow was already thick on the ground and still falling fast when I received the call at my home in Mottram, asking me to head up to their house in the Glossop hills, some three miles away. In situations like this it's standard practice to send an ambulance as well as two community midwives, in case it's too late to get the patient to hospital. One of my colleagues would also have had a call to provide me with back-up, though she was not here yet.

It was past 10 p.m. when my phone rang in my sitting room. I wasn't actually on duty, but as I drove a 4 x 4 and lived closest, I agreed to help. I must admit I wasn't entirely thrilled about this. My husband Peter and I were watching television and I had been feeling very cosy, cuddled up on the settee, drinking hot tea and warming my toes in front of the fire. We'd spent the evening wrapping presents and I'd baked a batch of mince pies, which filled our home with a wonderful festive smell.

'What a night to be called out,' I grumbled as I went to get changed into my uniform.

'Well, you won't be complaining about wearing trousers on a night like this, that's for sure,' Peter commented as he looked out at the wintry night.

He was right. In these conditions the only saving grace, if you could call it that, was that I no longer had to wear a dress to work. My NHS uniform had changed in 2000 to navy trousers and a matching cotton tunic, which I wasn't sure about at first. I remember that, not long before trousers came in, I'd been called out very urgently to a delivery, and for the first time ever I'd rushed out in my own clothes to save time changing. I found this was a big mistake. Even though the delivery went very well, I just didn't feel right at all.

Without my uniform I didn't actually feel like 'Linda the midwife'. I was just Linda, the person I am when I am off duty and, though I'm sure it didn't show, I felt somehow unprofessional. I vowed never to do that again, but when the modern trouser suit uniform was first unveiled I had my misgivings. It seemed so far removed from the days when I wore long skirts, starched cuffs and stockings and suspenders during my nurse's training in the 1960s, and I wondered if I would feel suitably attired and ready for action.

In fact, my fears were unfounded. The trousers proved to be very smart and practical, and on nights like this they were an absolute godsend.

A colleague at the hospital had informed me that Sarah had gone into labour with her first baby on her due date but had been too afraid to venture out in the snow, for fear of getting stuck and having to have the baby in the car.

I shivered as I stepped out onto my driveway, crisp new flakes of snow crunching under the soles of my black shoes. Peter always helped me start my car in the winter. He was a gem at times like this, and as he cleared the snow off the windscreen I began to check my A–Z as I didn't recognise the name of the road despite having worked in Glossop for many years. With this not being a scheduled home birth I had never visited Sarah before. I had not seen her at antenatal clinic, either, but that was not unusual as I typically shared a case load of about 80 ladies at any given time with the two other community midwives in my team, Helen and Angela. I realised as soon as I studied the route that I might have difficulty reaching the address, because it was in a remote part of Glossop, well off the beaten track.

As I navigated the near-empty roads taking me out of Mottram and towards Glossop, thick, icy snowflakes were bearing down on the windscreen of my Honda CRV. I had the heating on full blast, but I could still feel the bitter cold penetrating the fogged-up windows. It was 10.15 p.m. by now, and visibility was poor. Every road I drove down seemed to be darker and quieter than the last. The sky felt very low above me, crowding in on me as it deposited a relentless barrage of snowflakes on the roof of the car. Only the occasional flash of fairy lights blinking from a porch, or the twinkling of a Christmas tree in a window broke up the white landscape stretching and deepening around me.

I turned on the radio and was heartened to hear some Christmas carols tinkling out of the car speakers. I might have been reluctant to leave my warm and cosy house, but deep down I felt pleased to be helping a pregnant woman in her hour of need, sharing this precious night with her.

It took me about twenty minutes to reach Hathersage Drive, a main road on the east side of Glossop, which runs parallel to the picturesque Derbyshire Level and close to a golf course. I was used to seeing rolling hills and green grass from here, but everything was white except for the blue flashing light from a parked ambulance that now came into view.

Sarah's house was down a narrow lane leading off Hathersage Drive, but I knew as soon as I saw the ambulance parked up at the top of the lane that it was not possible to drive any closer. I pulled up behind the ambulance, had a quick word with the driver, who confirmed I was at the right address, and headed down the lane, delivery pack in hand.

I was wearing a jacket and gloves, and Peter had made sure I had my Wellington boots with me, but I hadn't expected to have to walk such a distance. It was several hundred yards down the lane and the snow was so deep in places that I could feel the cold and wet going down inside my boots and through my trousers. I'd never seen such deep snow, in fact, and I had to take big, wading strides to get through it. I wanted to phone ahead, but when I pressed the buttons on my mobile phone with my cold fingers, I found I had no signal.

More snow began to fall at this point, which stuck in my hair and coated my clothing. I gritted my teeth and ploughed on, telling myself I was very nearly there and to keep going. I was panting and breathless, and probably looked like a snowman when I finally reached Sarah's door.

The relieved and grateful look on Robin's face when he saw me standing there was one I had seen many times before. It didn't matter a jot that I looked like a snowman. I was a midwife underneath the snowflakes, and that was all the expectant dad could see in that moment.

Thank goodness Sarah had not delivered the baby before I arrived. This was not an ideal scenario, as Sarah had wanted to give birth in hospital, but as a community midwife I was well used to walking into situations where you simply had to make the best of things.

'Thank God,' Sarah blurted as soon as she saw me. She was wrapped in a pink cotton dressing gown and lying uncomfortably on the bathmat.

An ambulanceman was standing by, hovering beside the bathroom door. 'Well done. I think you've made it in the nick of time,' he said quietly to me as I dashed in and knelt at Sarah's side. As he spoke the patient let out a rip-roaring scream. 'Jesus Christ! It's killing me! Make it stop!'

I pulled on a pair of rubber gloves as hurriedly as I could, though my fingers were still numb with cold. 'I'm going to have a little look,' I told Sarah. 'Just keep breathing and panting as you are, that's good …'

'Jesus! Your hands are freezing!'

'I'm really sorry. But let's see … oh, that's good. You've done ever so well here.'

Water was trickling from my hair, leaving big wet blobs on Sarah's dressing gown. 'Sorry, again,' I apologised, wiping my face with the back of my forearm.

Sarah was ready to push, and I tried to soothe her with this good news. 'Just give me a moment while I get my instruments out. I'm going to tell you when to push, and I think your baby is going to be here very soon.'

'Will you hurry up?!' she said, which prompted her husband to let out an embarrassed laugh.

'There we are. Give me a nice big push right on your next breath … I can see baby's head. Lovely, lovely. You are doing really well …'

'Jesus. Jesus,' she cursed. Robin was holding one hand and Sarah thrashed about for something to grab hold of with the other. The nearest thing to hand was a toilet roll holder, which she squeezed for all it was worth.

Moments later I guided one small shoulder out, then the next. The atmosphere suddenly felt incredibly calm as the baby girl arrived very gracefully, slowly emerging into my hands. There was a brief moment of perfect silence in the room, and then the little girl let out a piercing cry. It was an absolutely beautiful delivery.

'There's nothing wrong with her lungs!' Robin gasped with relief.

'You can say that again. And she's not crying because I have cold hands,' I smiled. 'I've warmed up a bit now!'

Sarah burst into tears when she took hold of her baby daughter. 'Aren't you just perfect?' she told her. 'You're gorgeous!'

The new mum was propped up against the side of the bath by now, and someone had fetched a pillow for her to lean back on, but from the ecstatic expression on Sarah's face, any thoughts of being uncomfortable on the bathroom floor were not important right now. I could see snow falling outside the bathroom window, and the scene before me of mother and daughter sharing their first precious moments warmed my heart. This really was what life is all about.

Later, Sarah, baby Kate and proud new dad Robin invited me to sit with them around a roaring fire they had going in the lounge, which was decked out with a beautiful Christmas tree that filled the room with the smell of fresh pine needles. Robin made me a steaming mug of hot chocolate and we sat there chatting while I dried my clothes out. At about 2.30 a.m., when I was satisfied Sarah and Kate were both well, Robin drove me back down the lane in his Range Rover and made sure I could drive away safely, which, thankfully, I could. I had been told that the second midwife dispatched to the address had not made it through the snow and had had to turn back, so I was very grateful for Robin's help.

'Don't thank me,' he said. 'It's Sarah and I who are very grateful to *you*. I don't know what we would have done without you.'

I don't remember the cold or the bleakness all around me on my slow journey home. I was just thrilled to have played a part in Kate's safe arrival, and the adrenaline was still flowing through my body, all the way back to Mottram.

A decade on, I still have a very clear image in my mind of that brand new little family huddled together in front of the flickering fire. They looked a picture of happiness. Sarah's cheeks were flushed pink and she had a wonderful glow about her. Robin was beaming so brightly he practically had sparks of pride bouncing off him, and little Kate looked blissfully content, wrapped in a beautiful white fleece blanket as she slept soundly in her mother's arms.

It is one of the many births I will never forget in my forty-two years as a midwife. I have delivered more than 2,200 babies and I still have my heart in my mouth each and every time I report for duty. I never know what might take my breath away next, and that is why I continue to do the job I love.

Chapter One

'I'd love *to hear some good news'*

'Is there anything I can do to help, Nurse?

Mrs Sheridan's well-fed son Simon was fast asleep in the plastic cot beside her bed, and she could see that I was run off my feet on the busy new postnatal ward.

'Actually, yes, that's very kind of you,' I replied gratefully. 'Would you mind wheeling Tina in her pram?'

Baby Tina was a fragile little girl who had been born small for dates and was always hungry, which made her unsettled.

'It would be my pleasure,' Mrs Sheridan beamed. 'Poor little mite, I don't mind one bit.'

Baby Tina's mother was a seventeen-year-old girl who had decided to put her daughter up for adoption as soon as she was born. The young mother had discharged herself a few days earlier, leaving Tina in our care until the authorities were able to place her with a foster parent.

All the new mothers on this ward understood the situation, and a few had pitched in over the last day or two to give Tina a cuddle or a ride in her pram, whenever their own babies were sleeping soundly in their cots.

I directed Mrs Sheridan to the nursery, where Tina lay.

'Call one of the other midwives if Simon wakes up and you need to leave Tina, if she is not settled.'

'Don't worry, Nurse,' she smiled. 'I can manage, no bother.'

It was Thursday 3 February 1972, and local dignitaries were gathered downstairs, in the entrance to Ashton General Hospital's Maternity Unit, for the official opening ceremony. I had been told to try to attend the event, and so I slipped away, leaving the staff nurse in charge of the ward.

I quickly took the lift down to the ground floor, hoping to catch a glimpse of the historic moment when Sir John Peel, President of the International Federation of Obstetricians and Gynaecologists, would unveil a plaque on the wall, declaring the unit officially open.

I was a junior sister now and, as I stood at the back of the foyer that day, I allowed myself a moment of reflection and self-congratulation. My husband Graham, proud as ever, had bought me an antique silver buckle to attach to my red belt. I now wore a navy blue dress instead of a pale blue one and I had the 'frillies' on the cuffs of my short sleeves.

In becoming a sister in January 1972, one year after qualifying as a staff midwife, I had reached another milestone in my career. I felt a great sense of achievement as I watched the brass plaque being unveiled and listened to a succession of local dignitaries applauding our new 142-bed, £2 million maternity unit.

Sir John spoke of the tremendous advances in obstetrics, and of how modern techniques had combated the once high mortality rate amongst newborns. The Department of Health had achieved its national target of ensuring 70 per cent of births took place in hospital, he said, and in the Manchester

Hospital Region the figure exceeded 80 per cent. This meant that our new unit was much needed.

I smiled warmly as a beaming Mrs Randle, the mother of the first baby to be born in the new unit in December 1971, was presented with a silver cup while her son Jarrod slept in her arms, oblivious to his starring role in the proceedings. Lord Wright, Chairman of the Ashton and Hyde Hospital Management Committee, declared triumphantly: 'We are proud of this unit and we should take pride in seeing the happy, smiling faces of the mothers in the unit!' The local press turned out to cover the event and, as photographs were taken for posterity, I thought it was a day I would not forget.

Afterwards I returned to the postnatal ward with a real spring in my step. We had this whole five-storey unit all to ourselves, and I loved working in it. Gone were the days when the maternity unit was housed inside the old Ashton General Hospital. We still shared the same grounds, but now our new facility stood alone, a state-of-the-art 1970s steel-framed block, clad with contemporary concrete panels.

I'd excitedly watched the building work progress throughout 1970. I remembered peeping inside as the unit slowly began to take shape, excitedly imagining what it would be like to have ultra-modern plastic cots instead of old-fashioned cloth cribs, shiny store cupboards stocked with luxuries like disposable syringes and razors, and even paper caps and plastic aprons to replace our starched cotton ones. Now, I was actually working here – and as a junior ward sister, no less!

Stepping back inside the ward, I went straight over to Mrs Sheridan, who was rocking a very satisfied-looking Tina tenderly in her arms while her son Simon continued to sleep soundly in his cot. If Lord Wright were to walk in here now, I thought, he'd be delighted to see how well these new wards were working out, and he would indeed see the 'happy, smiling faces' he had talked so animatedly about. The atmosphere here was friendly, just as it was on the big open-plan Nightingale wards at the old maternity unit, yet there was a more intimate and peaceful feel to these smaller wards, too, as they were divided into rooms with four beds in each. I liked them very much.

'Good. You managed to settle her?' I said to Mrs Sheridan, who was looking very relaxed and had clearly had no trouble with either Tina or Simon.

'She did *ever* so well,' Mrs Sheridan replied, giving me a satisfied smile. 'Hope you don't mind, Nurse, but I gave her a little breastfeed.'

'Pardon?'

'Well, I knew it would be the only breastmilk she would ever get and I thought it would give her a good start. Simon's doing so well on my milk that Sister Kelly said she thinks I must be producing Gold Top!'

I gasped, feeling absolutely flabbergasted. Breastfeeding had gone out of fashion at the time, and was nowhere near as common as it is today – in fact, midwives had a job convincing most women of its benefits. The majority of women still asked for a course of Stilboestrol, prescribed to suppress their milk, and most opted to bottle-feed from day one. Mrs Sheridan was clearly not one of those women – far from it!

'Well, you've obviously done a very good job,' I said tactfully, taking a deep breath and lifting the contented baby girl out of her arms, my brain going into overdrive as I wondered how I was going to handle this one.

At that precise moment some of the dignitaries from the opening ceremony appeared in the corridor outside the ward.

Miss Sefton, Head of Midwifery, stood in the doorway and began enthusing loudly about the marvellous new facilities.

'Most of the accommodation is in four-bedded rooms which combine sociability with quietness,' I heard her say. 'And I am very pleased to say that the new unit is attracting the highest calibre of midwives. We are very proud of our staff – in fact Sister Buckley over there is the very midwife you may have seen on the posters advertising the new unit across the region …'

I took a deep breath and smiled over at them. I was normally very proud of the fact I was indeed the midwife who had been chosen to promote the new unit, and had had my photograph plastered all over Ashton and its surrounding area in the previous few months.

At that moment, however, I wanted the ground to swallow me up, and I was willing the entourage not to come any closer.

I can't describe how relieved I was when the assorted ladies and gentlemen smiled back approvingly and then continued their tour, walking away from me, down the corridor.

'Well, Mrs Sheridan,' I whispered, trying hard not to appear as flustered as I felt. 'Of course it's not really the done thing to breastfeed another woman's baby, but I know you have done it with the best of intentions. I shall have to tell Sister Kelly what you've done, though, I'm sure you'll understand.'

'I don't mind one bit,' she replied. 'Why would I?'

I look back today and am *still* flabbergasted; not simply by what Mrs Sheridan actually did, but by how much society has changed.

Nowadays, of course, no woman would dream of breastfeeding someone else's child like that. If she did, it wouldn't just be a question of informing the senior sister on the ward, who would most certainly not react in the way Sister Kelly did that day, which was to simply roll her eyes and say, 'I'll make a note, but there's no harm done, is there now?'

Blood tests would have to be carried out to make sure the baby had not been infected in any way, and the threat of legal action would be very real, but back then HIV was unheard of, and litigation was a word we rarely heard.

That said, what happened with Mrs Sheridan also reminds me how very *little* things have changed over the years. Mothers, and the depths of their maternal instincts, have never stopped amazing me, from that day to this.

About a month later, in March 1972, I was working a shift in the antenatal clinic when I saw a name I recognised – Mrs Sully – on my list. My gut reaction was that I was delighted to see this lady was pregnant again. In her case, I imagined those deep maternal instincts must have given her the strength and courage needed to try again, as she had lost her first baby in dreadful circumstances the previous summer.

I would never forget her arriving at the labour ward in the old hospital, brimming with hope and excitement, as she did throughout her pregnancy. I vividly remembered how every-thing had seemed so normal, until the awful moment I realised her baby's umbilical cord had prolapsed.

'There's something between my legs,' Mrs Sully had announced, setting off a heart-breaking chain of events. I had ridden beside Mrs Sully on the trolley as we dashed to theatre for an emergency Caesarean. I could see myself struggling to hold the baby's head back inside her, desperately trying to stop it crushing the escaped cord, which was hanging outside of the poor lady's body. I recalled seeing Mrs Sully struggling, too. She was thrashing about on the theatre bed instead of falling quickly asleep under the anaesthetic as we needed her to, in order for the surgeon to perform the Caesarean as quickly as possible.

I remembered the absolute chill that went through my body when I realised that Mrs Sully's baby son was born too late. He survived for just fifteen minutes, having been starved of oxygen in the womb. It was nobody's fault, just one of those exceptionally cruel twists of fate that occur so rarely, yet prompt you to wonder if there really is a God.

'I want a hatful of kids, I do,' Mrs Sully had said to me this time last year, the very first time I had met her in the old ante-natal clinic.

I had hoped and prayed that her wish would still come true despite her dreadful loss, and somehow I believed it would.

'Good morning, Nurse!' she smiled at me today.

I was delighted to see that the roses Mrs Sully had had in her cheeks when I first met her had returned. She was blooming again, cradling her tiny bump and looking as pleased as punch to be pregnant once more.

'Good morning, Mrs Sully,' I grinned back.

I was so relieved that she was still the positive and optimistic person I remembered. There was clearly no need for me to be apprehensive about seeing her again. Some women may have been reluctant – superstitious, even – to see the same midwife, but not Mrs Sully.

'I'm glad it's you,' she sighed, looking quite relieved. 'I was worried I might have to talk about what happened, go through everything again …'

I gave a little sigh of relief, too. As a midwife, if anything has not gone to plan, it's always a great comfort to know that the mother understands it was not your fault. Midwives are not miracle workers; we can only ever do our very best in the circumstances, and sometimes, sadly, that is just not good enough. Therefore, I was very glad to see that Mrs Sully was as happy to see me as I was to see her.

I examined Mrs Sully by palpating her abdomen and listening to her baby's heartbeat with a Pinard's stethoscope. Everything seemed in perfect order, and I was pleased to note that she was approximately sixteen weeks pregnant and her baby was due in late August. I was absolutely delighted for her; she certainly deserved some good fortune.

'That day,' she said wistfully. 'That day, I could never have imagined ever feeling happy again. Now it seems such a long time ago.'

'Doesn't it just,' I said, and we smiled at each other.

I had turned twenty-four a few days earlier, on 22 March 1972, and I felt more confident and self-assured than ever in my job. Being a ward sister made me walk just that little bit taller. It seemed such a long time ago that I had begun my training as a pupil midwife at Ashton General after three years of nurses' training at the Manchester Royal Infirmary. In fact it was just two years on, but so much had happened during my time as a midwife.

I remembered wondering, back in 1970, how I was going to manage to deliver forty babies – the required number for me to complete my ten-month training and qualify as a staff midwife. It had seemed such a huge number, but now it seemed so few.

In my first two years I had delivered over a hundred babies, and this new maternity unit seemed to be getting busier by the day as the Government continued to encourage women to have hospital births, believing them to be safer.

'I don't know about all this hospital birth business,' Mrs Tattersall, my community midwife mentor, had said to me on more than one occasion when I was learning the ropes from her as a pupil midwife out in the district.

'If you ask me, the best tools a midwife has are her hands. They're the same tools midwives have used since biblical times, and I have always thought you can't beat them.'

'Yes, Mrs Tattersall,' I agreed with her. 'But then again it's reassuring to have the paediatricians and doctors, and the theatre on hand if need be, sometimes.'

'Granted, Linda,' she said. 'But a good community midwife should be able to assess when a home birth is not a safe option. Look at it like this. If you give birth at home, there's a good chance you'll have two midwives attending – the community midwife and a pupil midwife. What happens in hospital? Tell me that? The place is always bursting at the seams, with one poor midwife trying to look after four or five labouring women all at the same time. Where's the sense in that? If you've got no complications, I can't see why any woman would choose to be stuck in hospital. That's a complication in itself, if you ask me.'

I was reminded of this conversation when I bumped into Mrs Tattersall in the car park when I was on my way into work one morning, in the spring of 1972. As usual she had a cigarette in one hand and delivery pack in the other, and she was rushing purposefully towards her trusty green Avenger.

'What a carry on!' she complained. 'What did I tell you about ruddy hospitals?'

'What's going on?' I asked.

'Flamin' laundry strike!' she retorted, charging past me. 'Can't stop. Third baby. Waters broke in the Co-op, would you believe.'

As soon as I arrived on the ward I was approached by an agitated Miss Sefton, who was carrying a bag of dirty baby linen. I was startled to see she was wearing a pair of green Wellington boots over her stockings instead of her usual small-heeled court shoes. The boots looked quite comical alongside her immaculately pressed Head of Midwifery uniform, but I tried not to react.

'Follow me, Sister Buckley!' she commanded.

Unfortunately, I think I must have gaped at her for a moment, as she chided: 'Don't just stand there, follow me!'

I did as I was told, and was amused to see she had turned the bathroom into a makeshift laundry and had been washing baby linen herself, in the bath.

'Please take over here,' she said. 'I have asked the patients to help us out and bring in their own linen and nappies where possible, but we simply cannot have dirty laundry littering the hospital. It is wholly unhygienic.'

'Right away,' I said, placing a disposable plastic apron over my uniform before I set to work.

'Thankfully we have managed to gain access to some twin tubs and dryers that are set up in another part of the hospital, but it's all hands to the pump I'm afraid,' Miss Sefton informed me.

The laundry workers' dispute lasted for about four weeks and the wards became more and more colourful by the day as patients brought in their own bed linen and baby clothes. Despite the newness of the wards, the only colour we were used to seeing was on the pretty floral curtains hanging around each bed. Cot sheets, blankets, bedclothes, nappies and baby nighties were all generally white or a very pale green, chosen to promote a tranquil environment on the ward.

Now, babies were dressed in pale pink, blue and yellow nighties and swaddled in blankets decorated with ducks, trains and goodness knows what else. One little girl even had a frilly lemon-coloured dress on, complete with tiny matching satin bloomers and a mob cap. The mishmash of colours made the wards look quite a muddle, but despite all this, the usual strict routines were adhered to.

For example, each lady was allowed just one or two congratulation cards and a vase of flowers on her locker top. There were never any giant teddy bears or bunches of balloons festooned around the beds as we have today; Miss Sefton would never have allowed such clutter.

'Come and sit with me and have a hot orange,' Sister Kelly said to me one morning, when order was finally restored. I can't remember much about the politics of the laundry workers' strike, but the workers certainly made the point that they provided a much-needed service which we could not manage without for very long. Trade union bosses secured the promise of improved pay and conditions for the workers, which hastened their return to work.

'Tell me, Linda, how are yer finding it here on Ward 29?' Sister Kelly asked.

I watched as she scratched her bosom through her uniform, the same way she had done on the first day I started at Ashton Hospital on 1 January 1970. I smiled to myself, thinking how much I enjoyed working alongside such a familiar character. I was no longer shocked by Sister Kelly's peculiar habits, and even when she wiped her nose on the back of her hand or wore the same tea-stained dress day after day, I didn't turn a hair.

'I absolutely love it,' I told her truthfully. 'I'm in my element here, I really am.'

'That's good, so it is,' she said. 'I'll let yer in on a secret. I had me doubts about the move, being that much older. But honest to God, I think it's marvellous here too, I really do.'

She sucked her teeth and looked me up and down.

'Tell me now, are you and that handsome husband of yours thinking of having babies of your own?'

'Oh yes, of course,' I said. I wasn't in the slightest bit put out by the question. I knew Sister Kelly liked any excuse to have a good chinwag, and this was friendly conversation, nothing more. Twenty-four was a very typical age for a young married woman to be starting a family, and it was something Graham and I were planning for in the very near future.

'Good for you,' Sister Kelly replied. 'I think having a baby yerself can only make yer an even better little midwife.'

I enjoyed talking to Sister Kelly. She was like a mother hen, and she always left me with a warm glow, whatever she said. I wasn't really sure that becoming a mother myself could make me a better midwife, and Sister Kelly herself was not a mother, but I nodded and enjoyed her friendly and supportive chatter all the same.

A few weeks later, at the beginning of May, I received an unexpected phone call from my father. 'Linda, your mum has a pain in her back and we're not going on holiday.'

My dad was always a man of few words, and on that occasion it turned out he excelled himself. The back pain was so severe my mum had been rushed into Ashton General to be checked over, and when I went in to visit her and find out what was going on she told me in a very matter-of-fact manner, 'I've had a heart attack.'

'What?!' I gasped. 'Dad told me you had a bad back.'

Mum looked perfectly fine, and a doctor appeared and explained that the heart attack had been very minor, and that she would be given drugs for angina and allowed home in a few days as long as she promised to rest.

'Has she been doing too much?' the doctor asked me.

'She works hard in our family bakery,' I explained.

'Perhaps it's time she took things a bit easier,' he suggested. 'She's been lucky this time, but this should be treated as a warning to her to slow down.'

'What a nuisance,' Mum said. 'I had my suitcase packed and everything.' That was typical of my mother. She has a fierce practical streak, and she has never been one to dwell on misfortune.

Mum was kept in for several days, and happily her recovery period was brightened up with the news that she had become a grandmother for the second time, which was a boost for the whole family.

My niece Tijen was born on 15 May 1972 in Vienna, a second child for my brother John and his wife Nevim, and a little sister for my twenty-month-old nephew Kerem. We couldn't wait to receive a photograph in the post, and when it finally arrived I was thrilled. Tijen looked very sweet, had dark hair and was very petite – a description that still fits her to this day, in fact.

We were all delighted, of course, and I think the new arrival, as well as the shock of suffering the heart attack, made my mother take stock of her life and put a few changes in place. She stopped work in Lawton's Confectioners, our family bakery, but was never one to sit around twiddling her thumbs, and so she took up pottery and painting. She was very good at both, but it wasn't enough for Mum. When she was fully recuperated a few months after the heart attack, she asked me if I might be able to find her a little job in the hospital.

'I can't just do that, Mum,' I said initially, not wanting to put myself in an awkward position with my employers.

'Please, Linda, love. Could you just ask the question?'

That was typical of my mum. She always said 'if you don't ask you don't get' and, even though I didn't always feel comfortable sharing that attitude, I admired my mum for practising what she preached. Reluctantly, I phoned the Assistant Matron's secretary, explained the situation and asked if there might possibly be any vacancies.

'Actually, yes there are, Sister Buckley,' came the reply. 'If your mother can come in for an interview this afternoon we may have just the job for her, but could she start soon?'

Mum couldn't believe her good fortune and hot-footed it to the hospital a few hours later, whereupon she secured herself a part-time post in the outpatients department of the main hospital, doing clerical work for the ECG patients. She was given a white tunic to wear and told to report for duty the very next morning.

'Thanks, Linda,' she said gratefully. 'It just goes to show …'

'If you don't ask you don't get?' I laughed. 'I thought you might say that.'

Still, I couldn't get over how incredibly lucky she had been with her timing. Something like that could never happen in this day and age. Jobs would never be given out to family members in such a way, and quite rightly so, but this was a different era and my mum certainly benefited from the old-fashioned way of things.

My parents lived in Ashton now and so Mum would even be able to walk to the hospital. Occasionally, we might be able to meet in the canteen for a cup of tea together if our shifts allowed. It seemed meant to be and, all things considered, I felt very blessed with my lot in life.

One afternoon I was sent to work on the antenatal ward as it was short-staffed. I didn't mind being moved around the wards; in fact I quite liked the change. I usually enjoyed the atmosphere on the antenatal ward. Expectation and excitement always hung in the air, yet there was typically a much calmer vibe than on the labour ward. The women here all had some sort of complication, warranting their stay in hospital before giving birth, which tempered their excitement a little.

It seemed quite peaceful today, despite the ward being full. There was a lady on bed rest who was expecting twins, and several women who were being monitored because they had high blood pressure. One woman, Beryl Johnson, was suffering from a severe chest infection and had been admitted earlier that day for observation and rest. She had the curtain pulled around her bed as she was coughing and spluttering, which made some of the other patients pass remarks.

'You'd think they'd have put her in a side room,' one woman said sympathetically.

'Maybe there isn't room,' another replied. 'Sounds like she's getting worse, though.'

The women generally didn't complain, but when they'd been confined to their beds for days or sometimes weeks, they would talk about anything and everything that came into their heads. You might hear them voicing opinions on the latest IRA atrocity or the Vietnam War one minute, swapping recipes or knitting patterns the next or debating whether the Osmonds or the Jackson Five were the best family singing group.

The most popular topic of conversation, of course, was always what had happened to other women they had met on the ward, who had now had their babies and left. At the start of this shift I gathered that a few weeks earlier a patient called Rowena had given birth to a very premature baby, as I heard one of the patients asking my colleague, Susan, how things were with that 'tiny little mite'.

'I couldn't believe my eyes,' I heard the patient say. 'What a shock it must have been for Rowena. She was such a lovely girl, too.'

'What exactly happened?' I asked Susan when we had a tea break. 'Oh, Linda, it was quite a drama,' Susan explained. 'I'm surprised this hasn't gone all over the hospital.'

She told me that Rowena had gone into premature labour at just 28 weeks.

'We were hoping the bed rest might stop things, but she suddenly pushed the baby out, totally without warning! It gave her such a terrible shock. She screamed hysterically, setting the whole ward into quite a panic.'

I dearly hoped the ending of the story was happy for Rowena and her baby, and I listened earnestly as Susan went on to tell me that Stella, a very competent new pupil midwife, was there in a flash.

'Honestly, you'd have thought she'd been doing this for years. Stella was ace. She wrapped the baby in a towel, tucked it down the front of her uniform and dashed across to Special Care, before you could blink.'

'And the baby survived?'

'Yes, he did!' Susan replied. 'It was a little boy. We heard he weighed just one pound, eight ounces, but he survived. Rowena has promised to pop in and keep us posted. Fingers crossed he's doing OK.'

This story inevitably reminded me of Muriel Turner, my patient at the old maternity unit whose premature baby appeared so frail and lifeless I thought he was dead, until he let out a very unexpected but very welcome cry. I relayed Muriel's story to Susan, explaining that I had carried the baby to the sluice, covered with a towel in a tiny bowl, thinking he hadn't made it.

'But he lived too, and he went home after about sixteen weeks,' I said. 'Let's hope Rowena's little boy proves to be just as much of a fighter.'

Muriel's story always gave me a good feeling and I never tired of telling it, especially in circumstances like this. In my mind, if Muriel's miracle baby could survive, there was hope for each and every premature baby, even this incredibly tiny one.

Returning from our break, Susan and I were alarmed to hear that Beryl Johnson's coughing had intensified quite significantly. Stella was on duty and looked extremely anxious as she stepped out through the curtain pulled around Mrs Johnson's bed.

'I've tried to make her as comfortable as possible,' Stella said. 'She's sitting in a chair and I've encouraged her to sip some water, but nothing seems to be working.'

It was at times like this that I was grateful for my nurses' training. Sometimes pregnant women are actually ill rather than suffering from a complication related to their condition, and I thought that perhaps an antenatal ward was not the best place for Mrs Johnson. She was thirty-six weeks pregnant, and the strain of coughing so vigorously must have been absolutely exhausting for her. She had been treated by her GP for repeated chest infections, but clearly none of the medication she had been given had managed to ease her chest or get the infection under control.

I offered to take over from Stella and found Mrs Johnson propped up uncomfortably in the chair, clutching her abdomen protectively each time her body choked out another wheezy, involuntary cough.

'I'm going to move you into a side ward and call the medical registrar,' I told her.

'Thank, huurgh huurrrgh th-thank you,' she spluttered.

The effort of speaking seemed tremendous. Mrs Johnson had bags under her eyes and not just dark circles but nearly black ones, and deep lines creased into her forehead. I saw from her notes she had recently turned thirty-five, but she looked ten years older. Her breathing was so laboured in-between coughs that she sounded like a person with severe asthma, and it was very apparent she needed more than the antenatal care we could give her on this ward.

Transferring her into a vacant side room along the corridor was difficult. Evelyn, a strong and capable auxiliary, helped me to guide Mrs Johnson into a wheelchair, but by now she was coughing so violently I was willing the medical registrar to arrive any second to take over the care of this patient.

'The doctor won't be long,' I reassured Mrs Johnson as I pushed the wheelchair as close to the window as possible, which Stella quickly opened.

'Don't try to talk, just concentrate on your breathing, help is on its way.'

She nodded gratefully but she had a frightened expression on her face every time she fought for breath, and she looked absolutely worn out. 'I'll leave her in the wheelchair for a minute or two before trying to move her,' I thought. I sincerely hoped her coughing wouldn't trigger contractions, as her lungs were in no fit state right now to support her through labour.

Suddenly Mrs Johnson's eyes flashed and rolled in her head.

'Th – ha – h – hurgh. Hurgh HURGHHHH' she spluttered, throwing her right hand up to her chest and slumping dramatically forward in the wheelchair.

My own heart tightened. I could scarcely believe it, but I knew exactly what was happening. Mine and Stella's startled eyes met temporarily. We both knew what to do and, drawing strength from a fear-loaded adrenaline surge, we manoeuvred Mrs Johnson onto the floor as quickly and carefully as possible. I started working on her chest and instructed Evelyn, the auxiliary, to run for help.

'Unless you ladder your stockings, to my mind you haven't made a good job of dealing with a cardiac arrest!' I could hear Sister Hyde's voice in my ear. That's what my old mentor had taught me on my very first day under her wing on the cardiac ward at the Manchester Royal Infirmary, and right here, right now, I was putting that training into practice with all my might.

Stella and I worked desperately on Mrs Johnson, giving her cardiac massage and mouth-to-mouth resuscitation. The medical registrar had arrived in the side room within moments, and he worked with us, offering words of encouragement as he did so. Stella had taken the same route as me into midwifery and was a newly qualified State Registered Nurse (SRN), and we worked well together.

My heart was pounding ten to the dozen as I worked on Mrs Johnson, but that did not stop my brain focusing on the job in hand and doing everything in my power to try to save my patient's life.

The crash team who deal with patients who have had a cardiac arrest arrived and took over the resuscitation. They began pushing down on Mrs Johnson's chest, trying to keep her heart beating, but the awful truth was starting to dawn.

Nothing seemed to be making any difference. It was one of those absolutely tragic situations where you are following all the correct procedures, doing the very best you can, but it is simply not enough. Mrs Johnson had had such a massive heart attack her life was possibly already lost before we started our desperate attempts to resuscitate her.

It wasn't until the moment when Stella and I looked across at the registrar, who gave the signal for everyone to stop trying to resuscitate Mrs Johnson and move away from the patient, that the enormity of what had happened began to hit me. This lady had died right in front of me, and her baby's life was lost, too. It was so horrendous the shock came over me in wave after wave.

I felt battered and wrung out. I tried to imagine Sister Hyde had been watching me, and that now she was reassuring me that I had done my very best, despite the unthinkable outcome.

I can't remember walking into the kitchen, but I know I sat very quietly alone in there with my thoughts for some time, drinking sweet tea. I felt the gentle hands of colleagues rubbing my back, and soft words being whispered around me. Nothing soothed my pain, however. I ached all over, and deep within my heart.

At around 5.30 p.m. Mr Johnson arrived at the hospital to see his wife. He had been ushered to sit in a side room by a rather nervous and unprepared female doctor called Dr Bodsworth, and I was called in, too. I looked at my watch and registered it was about half an hour since Mrs Johnson's death, though if someone had told me I had been sitting down in the kitchen for three minutes or three days I would have believed them. I absolutely dreaded seeing Mr Johnson and I had to peel my eyes off the ground to look at him as I entered the side room.

He was looking worried but not panic-stricken, and we greeted each other with a polite 'Hello.' Mr Johnson had clearly come straight from work. He was wearing a mechanic's boiler suit and still had traces of oil on his hands, though he smelled strongly of Swarfega, a heavy-duty cleaner he must have used hastily on his skin when he got the message to come to the hospital. I recognised the distinctive smell because Graham used it sometimes when he tinkered with his car.

'I'm sorry, but I have to tell you your wife has arrested,' Dr Bodsworth told Mr Johnson plainly.

'I see,' Mr Johnson said, nodding his head sagely but looking rather bemused. 'She'll be all right, though?'

'No, Mr Johnson, your wife has *arrested*,' Dr Bodsworth repeated, more slowly this time.

He looked to me, clearly not understanding the terminology.

'I'm very sorry, Mr Johnson, but your wife has died,' I said quietly.

The words seemed to hit him like a bullet in the stomach. His head dropped and he crumpled over in his seat and stared at the floor.

'The baby?' he asked eventually, looking up at me pitifully.

'The baby's died, too. I am so sorry.'

The three of us sat silently for what felt like an age until Mr Johnson asked, 'Can I see her?'

'Yes, of course,' I replied, glancing at Dr Bodsworth for approval. 'Come with me. She is in Room 2.'

Dr Bodsworth did not stop me, but she looked agitated. I had heard that she had questioned why no attempt had been made to deliver the baby, but I knew this was an inappropriate question to have asked, and nobody deigned to answer it. In the circumstances we had to try to save the mother first. That was correct medical procedure. We might have got Mrs Johnson's heart going and been able to perform an emergency Caesarean in the operating theatre, but it hadn't happened like that. We weren't to know what the outcome would be and we did what was required, swiftly and efficiently. Nobody was at fault. Nothing more could have been done, but nothing we had done had been enough.

'I'm very sorry about the baby,' I said to Mr Johnson, my voice cracking as we each took a seat beside his wife.

Mrs Johnson just looked as if she was sleeping, with the blanket pulled up over her chest and her arms flopped casually over the top of it. Mr Johnson squeezed his wife's left hand, smudging it with oil from his own hand.

'I wouldn't have wanted the baby without ... my Beryl,' he whispered, staring at the wedding band on her finger.

Noticing the oil mark he'd made on his wife's skin, Mr Johnson looked at her face and said apologetically, 'Sorry, love,' just as if she could hear him. I gulped and tried to stop the tears that were welling in my eyes from splashing down my cheeks, but I failed.

Mr Johnson tried to rub away the black mark from his wife's pale skin, but made it worse. 'What a mess,' he gasped, letting go of her and holding his head in his hands as he broke down. 'What a bloody mess.'

All these years on I still find it very difficult to revisit that day's events. I thought long and hard about whether to include Mrs Johnson's death in this book, but it did happen and so I decided I should. Her death was unusual in the extreme, however, and I certainly do not want to frighten anybody, particularly any pregnant women.

We found out from the post-mortem some weeks later that Mrs Johnson suffered from an extremely rare syndrome that affects blood pressure and heart rate and had unfortunately never been diagnosed. Her repeated chest infections most probably exacerbated her condition, but ultimately it was the little-known syndrome that killed her.

Even before the post-mortem results came back with that information I was sure in my own mind that Mrs Johnson's death was unrelated to her pregnancy. I desperately wanted to reassure the other women on the antenatal ward, who inevitably knew about the tragedy, and I chose my words carefully.

'Please don't worry yourself unnecessarily,' I told each and every one of them as the terrible news began to spread, setting off a very upsetting chorus of gasps and sobs. 'We do not know the exact cause of her death, but we do know that Mrs Johnson was not a well lady.'

I knew the women were all dreadfully sorry to hear the news, but a survival instinct kicks in with a pregnant woman, and the number-one priority is always her own baby, which she will protect at all costs. What these ladies desperately needed to know was that what killed Mrs Johnson was not going to strike them and their unborn child down, too. Even before the official cause of death was confirmed, I knew my message had to be that they and their baby were as safe as they were before Mrs Johnson ever arrived on the ward, which was the truth. It was right that they focused on that positive and didn't dwell on negative thoughts, because the alternative was unthinkable.

'So it wasn't the pregnancy that killed her?' several of the ladies asked me, one way or another.

'No, I believe not,' I replied. I smiled reassuringly at each pregnant lady and tried my hardest to put on a brave face, but inside I felt cold and sick.

'Thank goodness for that,' came the reply over and over again. 'What a terrible thing to have happened.'

At the end of my shift I sat in the kitchen alone, gathering my thoughts. Losing Mrs Johnson reminded me of other deaths I had encountered at the MRI, which I had found very difficult to cope with. Avoiding death is what led me into a career as a midwife. I wanted to bring new life into the world, not deal with illness and death, and now look what had happened. How *could* this have happened to Mrs Johnson and her baby?

'Linda, have you heard?' Stella said, breaking my thoughts.

I looked at her blankly.

'Have you heard about Rowena's baby?' she added. 'I thought you might like to hear some good news.'

I had to think for a moment before realising Stella was talking about the tiny premature baby she had carried to Special Care down the front of her uniform.

'I'd *love* to hear some good news,' I replied.

'He has gained two ounces already and is doing remarkably well. The milk bank's done him proud. Isn't that great?'

'It is,' I replied. 'It really is! Do the ladies on the ward know?'

She shook her head. 'Not yet.'

'Well, I think you should go and spread the news,' I smiled.

The milk bank was a stock of breastmilk collected from women on the wards who had a surplus after feeding their own baby. We got them to pump it into glass bottles so it could be used to feed the babies on Special Care, and it was always good to be able to tell other mums their milk was working its magic and helping another baby. The fact Rowena's fragile little boy was doing well was extremely uplifting, and just the news the whole ward needed.

Stella and I shared a look that told me she was thinking exactly the same thoughts as me. It's an emotional rollercoaster, working as a midwife. You just never know when you might be plunged into a dark abyss, or when you may be launched back up into the bright sky. As I prepared to leave for the day it was very heartening to hear a succession of 'oohs' and 'aaahs' filling the ward as news of Rowena's baby travelled fast.

I thought that Stella seemed to have coped with Mrs Johnson's death well, perhaps better than I had. She had dried her eyes quickly and got on with the job in hand, looking after the other patients on the antenatal ward efficiently yet compassionately.

I wondered if it was because she had finished her nurses' training so very recently, whereas I was far less used to dealing with death nowadays. Thank God I had become a midwife, I thought. Thank God that tomorrow I would be back on the postnatal ward, where I would have the honour and joy of helping to care for a brand new life.

Chapter Two

'Please God, look after Mrs Sully this time'

I had an unsettling sense of *déjà vu* when I began work on the postnatal ward one warm and sunny morning in July 1972.

There was a new arrival in bed one: a raven-haired lady who was wearing a beautiful bat-wing nightgown made of a lovely blue chiffon material. She had a neat little chignon pinned into the back of her shoulder-length hair and she had clearly spent quite a bit of time applying her make-up, which was practically unheard of for a tired new mum. Her eyebrows were pencilled in dark kohl, her sharp cheekbones were highlighted with a dark rouge and she was wearing fetching coral-coloured lipstick, which I'd read in a magazine was the height of fashion.

'Good morning,' I said brightly, scanning the notes as I approached her bed. 'I see you've had a lovely little boy Mrs Prince, congratulations! Phillip's a lovely name.'

Beneath the blusher, I was confused to see the colour suddenly and completely drain from Mrs Prince's face, and I asked her if she was feeling all right.

'I'm fine,' she mumbled, lowering her eyes shyly and putting one hand up on her brow, as if shielding her face from the sunlight shining through the window. 'Everything is perfect. I think I'll get some sleep, whilst Phillip is settled.'

I knew Mrs Prince was an accountant by trade, as one of my colleagues had mentioned it in passing. I had started to notice that the more educated the woman, the more pressure she put herself under to be the perfect mother and the perfect wife. I wondered fleetingly if perhaps Mrs Prince was one of those high-achieving people who had to have everything 'just so'. That would certainly explain her fine appearance.

I left her in peace, closing the curtain around her bed, and went about my duties on the ward. I chatted to several women about how much milk their little one had taken, whether the baby's umbilical cord was drying up nicely or how uncomfortable the new mother's stitches were.

There was a little alarm bell ringing in my head all morning, though, and I started to wonder if I had seen Mrs Prince before. I thought I might have done, but I just couldn't place her. I would keep an extra eye on her today, as there was something about her I just couldn't put my finger on.

The three other new mums in this room on the postnatal ward were chatting easily to each other, discussing the latest plot on the television soap opera *Crossroads* and giggling about a well-thumbed copy of *Cosmopolitan* magazine one of them had picked up in the day room.

'I don't think my Barry would agree with this!' Mrs Vaughan snorted.

I could see she was holding the first-ever issue of the women's glossy magazine *Cosmopolitan*, as I'd flicked through it myself one day in a spare moment. It had caused quite a stir when it was published several months earlier, in March 1972, as it was far more outspoken and controversial than any of the other women's magazines available at that time.

'Listen up, ladies,' Mrs Vaughan chuckled as she began to read out one of the headlines on the bright red cover. '"An extraordinary interview: Michael Parkinson talks about his vasectomy – the most beautiful thing a man can do for a woman."'

All three women fell about laughing, clutching their abdomens and wincing as they did so.

'And there's me having me tubes tied on Friday!' hooted Mrs Rogers from the bed opposite.

It was very common in those days for women who had completed their family to stay in hospital and have a Pomeroy sterilisation under general anaesthetic approximately five days after giving birth. It means having an abdominal incision and both fallopian tubes clamped, cut and tied to prevent future pregnancies. Doctors carried out at least half a dozen each week, if not more, which was part of the reason the postnatal wards were always full.

Condoms, often referred to as 'Johnnies', were the other preferred choice of contraception at that time, although many couples tried to manage without and lived in fear of unwanted pregnancy, as you still had to pay for the Pill back then. It was typical for married women, rather than their husbands, to take responsibility for sterilisation. Very few men were as enlightened as Michael Parkinson when it came to vasectomies, I think it's fair to say.

'Well, I wish Parky would tell that to my Eddie,' chipped in Mrs Griffiths, who had just given birth to her second child. 'I'd certainly consider it a beautiful thing if he had the snip!'

To a choir of approving noises, Mrs Griffiths went on to complain that it was far easier for a man to have a vasectomy than for women to be sterilised. 'It's a tiny op for them by comparison, for goodness sake! If you ask me, we've done our bit by giving birth. Going under the knife is beyond the call of duty!'

The other women were in wholehearted agreement, including Mrs Rogers, who was already booked in for the operation. 'You're right, love,' Mrs Rogers said wistfully. 'But by the time I'd argued that one with my husband I'd probably be in the family way again. I'll not be taking any more chances.'

With that the conversation shifted to the next headline. It was something about 'How to turn a man on when he's having problems in bed.' This set off a predictable chorus of groans and remarks like: 'No thanks – I'm done with all that for the time being, thank you very much!' and 'I'd rather learn how to turn him *off*!'

Mrs Prince remained very quiet, keeping herself to herself behind her drawn curtain while all of this banter was going on. I made a mental note to check her previous notes when I got the chance, in case that might enlighten me. The more I thought about it, the more I was convinced I'd seen her before, somewhere else in the hospital perhaps.

At visiting time I wondered if seeing her husband might trigger my memory, but when Mr Prince arrived with an extravagant bunch of carnations, I definitely had no recollection of ever having seen him before.

'Congratulations, Mr Prince,' I said, having a good look at him. He was wearing some expensive-looking velvet bell-bottom trousers and appeared extremely well to do.

'Your son is doing well, I'm glad to see,' I remarked, hoping to engage him in conversation.

'Thank you very much indeed, Nurse,' he said politely. He looked thoroughly smitten as he peered in Phillip's cot as his wife sat silently in bed, watching a little nervously.

'I don't mind admitting that I really wanted a son and heir, and I'm so pleased! I've got two weeks off work to get to know him, too. I couldn't be happier!'

'Well, I'm very pleased for you …'

Mrs Prince interrupted our little chat, asking her husband to keep the curtain drawn and telling him she felt tired and wanted peace and quiet. She looked tense and very serious, and kept her eye gaze down.

'Of course you need to rest, darling,' he said, kissing her gently on the forehead. 'Look at you – immaculate as ever despite having just given birth … can I go and fetch you anything from the shop?'

I was still none the wiser, and so I dug out Mrs Prince's file as soon as visiting was over. Scanning her most recent notes, nothing gave me a clue, although of course in those days we only kept written copies that were certainly not as lengthy as the computerised patient records we have today.

I saw that the couple lived at a smart address in Broadbottom. Mrs Prince had no health problems and her pregnancy and delivery had been completely routine. Looking further back, my eyes bulged as they fell on a brief page of notes dated February 1971, which were fastened at the back of this thin brown file. Mrs Prince had delivered a healthy baby boy more than a year ago and, according to a very scant note, had given the child up for adoption at birth. The handwriting was difficult to read, but the words 'Social Services' leaped out, telling me the local authority had organised the adoption.

My brain whirled. That's why I recognised Mrs Prince! Last year, I had seen her at the old hospital. She had attended an antenatal appointment alone, dressed smartly in a business suit and constantly looking at her watch, worrying about getting back to her desk before her lunch hour was over, or at least that's what she told me. Her hair was longer then and her make-up was different, but this was definitely one and the same person. Racking my brain, I recalled how she had told me that her husband was away working, on the oil rigs.

It was all coming back to me now, though I could hardly believe it. When Mrs Prince went on to give the baby up for adoption I remembered how it came as a real surprise to all the midwives on duty, as this had not been discussed at all during her pregnancy. My mind was in overdrive as I fished for more memories to help piece this puzzle together. I was sure Mrs Prince had told a colleague that she intended to go back to work straightaway. Her husband was not ready to start a family, and she did not want a child to disrupt her career, that's the story she told when she made her surprise announcement about the adoption.

At the time, her explanation didn't seem to ring true and rumours abounded. I remembered the gossip in the office one day. Was there actually a husband working away on the oil rigs, and if there was, did he even know about this baby?

'It's my betting this is a secret love child,' my colleague Maggie had said to me back then, eyes widening.

I wasn't convinced. 'Maybe it *is* her husband's baby and she just doesn't want to tell him, because she's the one who's not ready to start a family yet,' I had replied.

Both scenarios were as difficult to believe as Mrs Prince's own story about the adoption, and I remembered feeling resigned to never knowing the truth.

Now, I felt compelled to confide in Sister Kelly. I took a deep breath and walked into her office.

'I-I need to talk to you,' I stuttered. Sister Kelly put down her mug of Bovril and was all ears.

'I recognise Mrs Prince, and Phillip is not her first baby,' I blurted, feeling instantly relieved at having shared the burden of my discovery.

'Well my dear, yer never fail to be surprised in this business,' Sister Kelly shrugged, peering at the notes I thrust at her. Mrs Prince clearly hadn't lied on paper, as all her previous records were intact and tallied with everything we knew of her. It was only here, on this postnatal ward, that she had tried to cover up the fact she'd had a previous baby.

I explained all this to a rather bemused looking Sister Kelly, and concluded that Mrs Prince must have succeeded in keeping her poor husband away from her recent antenatal appointments as well as Phillip's delivery, which was not a difficult feat in 1972.

'But it's no wonder she is so tense here on the ward, trying to keep such an enormous secret!' I said.

Really, it had not been rocket science to piece together her full history. Any of the midwives, even if they hadn't recognised her as I had, could have stumbled across this information. I was astonished she had the nerve to try to pull this off at all, but Sister Kelly hardly turned a hair.

'It's really none of our business now, is it, Linda?' she sighed. 'I mean, if a woman turns up on the postnatal ward and tells you this is her first pregnancy, why would you doubt her? If it were me, mind, I think I'd have gone to a different hospital, but it takes all sorts.'

'But ... how could she?' I asked. I was completely nonplussed. 'Surely he should know, Mr Prince, whether the other child was his or not?'

'Well, Linda, when you look at Mr Prince, happy as a sand boy as he clearly is, what would be gained from spilling the beans now? Tell me that.'

'Nothing, I suppose,' I replied resignedly.

'That's right,' Sister Kelly said, shoving her hand down her dress and repositioning her bosom matter-of-factly, as if to show me everything was back to normal. 'Nothing at all! Put it to the back of your mind, dear. Now, would you like a hot orange?'

'No, thanks,' I said. 'I could probably do with something stronger, but a good cup of well-brewed tea will do fine!'

I'm sure I'd been refusing Sister Kelly's offer of hot orange for two years now, but she never failed to offer it to me when she felt I needed looking after. I've no idea why. I completed my shift that day, going through the motions of carrying out all my usual jobs on the ward, but I couldn't get Mr and Mrs Prince out of my head.

'Have you been to the bathroom?' I asked several ladies in turn, just as I always did. 'Let me have a little feel, make sure your uterus has contracted as it should ... now then, have you got any pains in your legs?'

The routine postnatal checks were second nature to me, which was just as well as I felt quite distracted. I just couldn't stop wondering how people could live such complicated lives. How did people get themselves into such a muddle? I couldn't help reflecting on the very sad case of Mrs Johnson, too.

Terrible things happened to people; tragic events beyond anybody's control. So why do others choose to go down a difficult path, all of their own accord?

I thought about my own life, and not for the first time I thanked my lucky stars for the hand I'd been dealt. I couldn't have asked for a better start. My parents always wanted the very best for me, and fortunately had the means to send me to a private school. It was strict at Harrytown High School, being educated by straight-laced nuns, but as an adult I could see how it had given me a good, solid foundation in life.

If it wasn't for the high expectations the headmistress Sister Mary Francis had for me, I would never have applied to do my nurses' training at the prestigious MRI. I was very glad I did, even though it was extremely tough. I would not be here today if I hadn't worked as hard as I did, passing my exams and gaining a pupil midwife place at Ashton General.

'Let's have a look at baby's cord ... shall we give baby a little top and tail, as I see she has some white stuff under her arms? Don't worry, it's just the waxy vernix that's been protecting her in the womb, a little wash will sort that out.'

I'd said the same things countless times on this ward, but on this day I couldn't help worrying that little bit more about each mother and her baby. I looked at them and hoped everything was as normal as it seemed, and if it was, I wished Mrs Prince could be just like them. How awful it must have been for her, living with such a lie, not to mention having to see me on the ward, an uncomfortable reminder of the past. She clearly remembered me, and for all she knew I could blow her whole world apart in an instant with an ill-timed recollection.

I wanted to reassure Mrs Prince that her secret was safe with me, but I certainly didn't want to cause her any more stress, so I just kept quiet. Towards the end of my shift I diligently asked Mrs Prince if she wanted to join some of the other ladies in the nursery for a baby-bath demonstration, or whether she needed any help at all with little Phillip's feeds. The answer was a firm but polite 'no' to both, as I thought it would be.

I think I was as relieved as Mrs Prince herself when she was discharged forty-eight hours after giving birth, which was typical then, provided there were no complications. I happened to be in the car park, just arriving for work in my electric blue Volkswagen Beetle – my pride and joy at that time – when I saw Mr Prince proudly carrying Phillip out of the hospital in a Silver Cross carrycot. He placed the carrycot carefully on the back seat of a brand new BMW as a smiling Mrs Prince looked on. I silently wished them all the best, hoping they could go on and live a happy life together.

My life seemed so very simple by comparison to theirs. I was just seventeen when I met Graham, and we married when I was twenty-one. Now, after seven years together, we were on the cusp of starting our own family. We'd talked about it excitedly for months, and had recently decided to stop taking precautions. As we were already in July by now, I calculated that even if I caught quickly I would have worked for more than a year as a junior sister before I might be taking maternity leave in 1973. I had it all worked out, and I was very grateful to have not only had such a solid, comfortable start in life, but to have landed on my feet in a loving marriage, where we had no secrets from one another.

* * *

September 1972 proved to be a very busy month. 'All dem Christmas parties!' Sister Kelly commented, referring to the fact that September, being nine months after the Christmas party season, is traditionally the busiest month on the maternity unit.

'Yer hear the same thing every year,' she lamented. 'Forgot the Pill. Threw up because of the drink. Honest to God, it's the same story year in, year out. Will these women never learn?'

I had to smile at her reference to 'the drink', because it was well known that Sister Kelly herself liked a little tipple from time to time, when she was off duty.

One morning I was dispatched to the labour ward, as it was 'bustin' at the seams' according to Sister Kelly. 'They need an extra pair of hands, so they do. It's like a conveyor belt in those delivery rooms.'

I was pleased to see Sister Judith Houghton on duty. I'd had a soft spot for Sister Houghton ever since she helped me deliver my very first baby as a pupil midwife, and every time I saw her I remembered the warmth of that first baby's head in my hands. It never failed to thrill me, and I was delighted to be with her on the labour ward today.

'We have Mrs Sully on her way in,' Sister Houghton told me as she allocated the jobs.

My heart jumped on hearing that name. Just as when I'd seen Mrs Sully at antenatal clinic back in March, I had a somewhat mixed reaction to seeing her again. I was absolutely thrilled that she was having another baby after losing her first so tragically, but I was also very anxious that nothing should go wrong this time round. 'She'll be here any minute.'

Sister Houghton explained to me that Dr Bedford, one of our consultants, had kept a very close eye on Mrs Sully in recent months. She was slightly overdue but there was nothing whatsoever to indicate she might suffer complications this time round, as the prolapsed cord that proved so calamitous last time was caused, very cruelly, by extreme bad luck.

'Would you like to take care of her?' Sister Houghton asked.

'Of course,' I replied without hesitation. 'I'd be very pleased to.' I meant it, and Sister Houghton gave me a knowing smile. When a mother has lost a baby as Mrs Sully did, there is nothing the midwives want more than to see her return and deliver a healthy baby. Sister Houghton knew very well that I had been deeply affected by Mrs Sully's loss, and she knew how much it would mean to me to deliver her baby this time round.

I took a moment to compose myself in the office. 'Please God, look after Mrs Sully this time,' I said silently.

I pulled my shoulders back and held my head high. I wanted everything to run smoothly for Mrs Sully, I really did. When she arrived on the ward, escorted by her husband, I was pleased to see she looked radiant and remarkably calm. Her face lit up when she saw me.

'It's good to see a familiar face, I'm pleased it's you,' she smiled, hands linked protectively underneath her extremely large bump.

'I'm pleased, too,' I replied. I had been prepared to step aside should Mrs Sully have wished, and I was very glad that was not necessary.

Taking careful steps and supported by her attentive husband, Mrs Sully went into the first-stage room.

'This is Malcolm,' she said. 'He's staying with me all the way through.'

I was glad to hear that. It was still quite uncommon for men to accompany their wife during the delivery, but if we thought they might help in any way, most midwives had started to encourage the men to consider it. The majority of expectant fathers refused, but recently I'd started to notice a very slight shift, with a few more men shuffling in to the delivery rooms. In my experience, the trick was to suggest they would have an important job to do.

'I think it would help your wife if you could rub her back,' I might say, or, 'Your wife is a little anxious; perhaps if you held her hand and talked to her you might be able to keep her calm … There's no need for you to be at the other end of the bed – unless you want to be, that is …'

I never put pressure on men to attend, but if I thought their wife might gain some comfort or benefit from it, I tried to encourage it. In Mrs Sully's case, I suspected her husband would be a great support and I was glad the decision was already made. He was an impressively tall and strong-looking man, and he appeared as calm and good-tempered as his wife.

'I work in the labs at Manchester University,' he said confidently. 'Don't worry about me, I am used to blood and that kind of thing.'

At that precise moment a woman in the neighbouring delivery room let out a blood-curdling cry, followed by a string of expletives.

'Don't you bloody well touch me!' she shrieked, presumably to the poor midwife. 'And ya can tell that fella of mine the same, wherever he is! I don't want him near me EVER again! I NEVER want to have another kid! Aaaargghhhhh! Arrrghhhhh! Bleedin' hell. Make it stop NOW! Why don't the men have to do owt? Why is it all left to US? Aaaaarghhhh!'

'I'm sorry you've had to hear that,' I said apologetically. 'But I'm afraid we do hear quite a lot of effing and jeffing in here.'

To my surprise and relief, Mr and Mrs Sully both started to laugh.

'Effing and jeffing!' Mr Sully said. 'I've not heard that expression before. It's really funny!'

'Have you not? I say it all the time. I think it sums up the nonsense we have to hear sometimes quite well!'

With the ice broken, I felt comfortable enough to ask Mrs Sully to go to the bathroom and produce a urine sample. This, we all knew, was the point where things had started to go so dreadfully wrong last time, but Mrs Sully did not make a drama. Her husband helped her into the adjoining toilet and stood guarding the door, and a couple of minutes later the process was completed.

All was well with the sample, and I helped Mrs Sully up onto the bed for an internal examination. This was all going to plan, I was sure. I must admit, though, it was still a relief when I saw with my own eyes that nothing untoward was happening down below. I felt my shoulders relax ever so slightly inside my dress as I noted that Mrs Sully was doing very nicely indeed, and was already four centimetres dilated.

'Thank you, Nurse,' she said to me kindly when I told her she was progressing well. 'I wasn't looking forward to that bit at all, but I'm fine. Can I just ask one thing? Would it be all right if I didn't have a shave and all that? It's just that with Malcolm here …'

'Of course!' I replied. 'Honestly, not long ago the Senior Sister would have asked questions if we didn't stick to those routines, but things are starting to change, I'm glad to say. It's not so strict any more.'

Mrs Sully looked visibly relieved, and I thought how ridiculous it was that any woman should have to worry about such things as a shave and enema at a time like this. I'd always been a bit dubious about the benefits of shaving a woman in labour anyhow. As for enemas, well, let's just say if nature required the bowels to be emptied, in my opinion usually the woman could manage this without the aid of soapy water being administered up her rectum in the 'high, hot and a hell of a lot' fashion I had been taught in the Sixties.

It was another three hours before Mrs Sully was fully dilated and ready to push. Because of her previous obstetric history, Dr Bedford had stepped into the delivery room and the theatre staff were alerted and kept informed of her progress throughout. Mr Sully held his wife's hand tightly as her contractions made her groan and shake her head from side to side on the pillow.

'You are doing absolutely brilliantly,' I said. 'Do you think you can give me one big push, when I tell you?'

'Ye–yeeessssss,' she moaned, biting her lips and wrinkling her brow.

I could see the head now, and I knew this baby was tantalisingly close to being delivered. Mrs Sully gripped her husband's hand so hard she made him yelp like a puppy as she gave an almighty push, exactly when I wanted her to. To my surprise the baby, complete with a thick mop of black hair, practically shot out in one fell swoop. Mrs Sully had delivered him with such force and determination that if I hadn't been ready to catch him, he might have shot clean off the end of the bed.

'It's a little boy,' I declared breathlessly as the red-faced baby let out an ear-splitting cry. His head appeared slightly squashed, which was very normal, but apart from that he appeared to be perfectly healthy.

'Congratulations!' I said, tears leaking down my cheeks. 'Well done to you both!'

I looked at Mrs Sully and saw that she was sobbing and laughing all at once.

'I've done it!' she said, sounding triumphant and ecstatic despite being completely exhausted. 'Can I hold him?'

'Any minute now,' I said as I swiftly cut and clamped the cord with trembling hands.

It had been such a high-speed delivery I was throbbing with adrenaline. As I cleaned and weighed the baby as quickly as possible, I suddenly realised Mr Sully had been very quiet. I glanced to where I expected him to be, standing at the side of the bed, and was puzzled to see him sitting in a chair by the window, his head between his legs. Dr Bedford, whose intervention had thankfully not been required during the delivery, was standing over him, which was a very unexpected turn of events indeed.

'There, there, my good man,' Dr Bedford was saying. 'Stay seated, I will get a nurse to attend to you.'

To my amusement I learned that, despite working with blood samples in the university laboratories, Mr Sully had passed out momentarily when he witnessed his son's dramatic arrival into the world. Dr Bedford's medical skills may not have been necessary during the birth, but the consultant's swift reactions meant that he spotted that Mr Sully was about to faint, and had steered him expertly into a chair, no doubt preventing him from cracking his head on the floor.

'Malcolm!' Mrs Sully exclaimed when she realised what had happened. 'You daft 'apeth! We've got a little boy! We've got a little boy! And he's all right!'

Mrs Sully was holding her son in a blanket by now. By this time there was another doctor, a paediatrician and another midwife as well as myself and Dr Bedford in the room, and Mrs Sully's joyful words set everyone off with wobbling lips and tear-filled eyes. We all took it in turns to congratulate the beaming new mum and take in the wonderful scene. My legs felt like jelly, and I imagined us all standing like dominoes, about to tumble around the bed because our bodies were quivering with so much emotion. It was a day I will never forget.

Chapter Three

'W-w-what did I do wrong?'

'I have some news, I think,' I told Graham one morning.

He raised an eyebrow and looked up from his cornflakes to see me standing there in my uniform with both hands laid gently on my belly.

'I think this is it. I think I'm pregnant!'

Graham's face shone instantly. He could not have looked happier if he tried, and he asked me a string of questions about when we would know for sure, how many weeks I might be and when the baby would arrive.

It was June 1973 and Graham and I had been trying for our own baby for several months. I had been a sister for more than twelve months, which was an achievement I had wanted to get under my belt before having a baby of my own. Everything was just as I'd planned.

'Has your job ever put you off having your own children?' my old friend Sue Smith had asked me one night when we were catching up on the telephone.

She worked as a schoolteacher in South Wales now and had a baby daughter called Miranda, and I think my reply was something along the lines of, 'I suppose I could ask you the same thing!'

If was a fair question from Sue, I suppose, and one that I'd been asked several times before in recent years. Never once did

I take it very seriously, though. The fact that I'd seen some very sad outcomes, not to mention having witnessed women suffering terribly in labour, never put me off wanting to have children of my own.

It was very unusual for things to go badly wrong, and when Graham and I had made the decision to start a family I was filled with nothing but optimism and hope about becoming a mum. In fact, I thought nothing could go wrong for me at all, which may seem a little unbelievable, but it was true. The hundreds of joyful births, the wonderful, heart-warming deliveries I'd been a part of and the love-filled faces of the new mums – that was what I thought of, and that was what I envisaged for myself.

When I suspected that I actually was pregnant, I could not have felt happier.

'The GP will have to send a urine sample off for testing,' I told Graham. 'I'll make an appointment today. Then it could take a week or so to get the result.'

'A week or so? Couldn't you find out sooner, through work?'

'I'll try,' I replied. 'Leave it with me.'

You couldn't just buy pregnancy kits at the chemist in those days, and we midwives inevitably saw it as a perk of the job to be able to use our skills to help each other out. I was back on the labour ward with Judith Houghton at this time, and I waited until I had the chance to take her to one side.

'I think I'm pregnant,' I whispered excitedly. 'Would you have a little listen for me?'

'Of course! How wonderful, Linda,' she replied. 'We could nip off and do it now if you like. Let me get hold of a monitor.'

We entered an empty side room where Judith listened to my abdomen using a hand-held foetal heartbeat monitor called a Sonicaid. These were quite new to the hospital and were in fairly short supply, and the early models were a little temperamental to operate. This meant the old-fashioned Pinard's stethoscope was still more commonly used, and we typically only used a Sonicaid on patients who had experienced a bleed or gone into premature labour. However, amongst ourselves it was viewed as quite an exciting perk of the job to use the Sonicaid on each other.

'I think these things are wonderful,' Judith commented as I lay on the bed and unbuttoned the front of my dress while she swiftly switched on the monitor. She slid the head of the plastic device over some jelly applied to my tummy, and moments later the Sonicaid's ultrasound waves picked up a heartbeat. We both squealed excitedly.

'I think your diagnosis may be correct,' Judith said giving me a hug 'Congratulations, Linda.'

I knew that the Sonicaid generally only picked up a heartbeat from ten weeks, or more likely twelve, which tied in with my dates. I would have to wait for a referral from my GP, of course, before I could book myself into the antenatal clinic and announce the good news publicly, but in that moment I had a very good idea that if my calculations were correct, by January 1974 I would be a mum, and I was thrilled to bits.

Looking around the labour ward later that same day, I had a sense of feeling slightly more connected to the women than I ever had before. I saw them as kindred spirits as well as patients now, and I looked forward to being able to confide in my patients, and tell them that I too had a new life inside me. I was having a baby, just like them.

'I hope you'll set a good example,' Judith teased when we went on a tea break later. I'd told her I wanted to have my baby here at the maternity unit, as I knew I would be well looked after and would feel comfortable in such familiar surroundings. It never entered my head to go anywhere else, in fact. Why would it?

I also hoped very much that Judith might be able to deliver me, although I knew very well that you could never be certain who your midwife would be, not just because of shift patterns but because of the uncertainty of delivering on your due date.

'I'll be a model patient, I promise!' I laughed. 'Can you really imagine *me* hollering like some of the ladies we see on the ward?'

'No!' Judith retorted. 'I don't suppose I can, but you never know!'

Several weeks later, after my pregnancy had been officially confirmed by my GP, I attended my first antenatal appointment. Graham was even more excited than I was about the baby, if that were possible, and offered to take time off work to come with me. It was still very uncommon for men to come into the clinic, however. Also, my colleagues were very good to me and always slotted me in when I was on duty and could pop in during a break.

'There's really no need to come,' I told Graham. 'I'm perfectly fine on my own. You stay at work, you've got a lot on.'

'Whatever you say, Linda,' he replied. 'You're the expert here.'

Graham's vending supplies business was doing well, and he and his brother had expanded it and moved into new premises. It was lovely that he wanted to support me every step of the way, but we both knew there was really no necessity, and the business needed him more than I did.

I'd grown up an awful lot in the time I had known Graham. Gone were the days when I relied on him to hold my hand and dry my tears after a tough day, as he did so many times when I was a teenager during my training at the MRI. I was a much more independent person now and, of course, when it came to having babies I was indeed the expert.

I asked if I could have Dr Bedford as my consultant as I had always admired his skills and his extremely pleasant bedside manner. My 'booking in' appointment was completely routine. I had no problems to report, and Valerie, the midwife in the clinic, listened to the baby's heartbeat with the Sonicaid, which of course was so lovely to hear again. She also confirmed what I had already worked out myself, that my due date was 7 January 1974. It felt a little odd sitting on the other side of the desk, but it wasn't unusual for midwives who worked at Ashton to have their babies in the maternity unit, and I felt at ease.

I returned to the labour ward feeling on top of the world, and looking forward to sharing my exciting news with all of my colleagues. However, I was dismayed to discover something of a staff meeting going on in a side room, where several midwives were assembled with Sister Margaret Penman, who was looking very serious.

'Do come and join us, Sister Buckley,' she called when she spotted me. 'We're just discussing the supplies being ordered on the night shift. You may have something to add.'

I walked in to hear Sister Penman, who was the senior sister on the labour ward, explaining very seriously that an unprecedented amount of flour, bicarbonate of soda and butter had been ordered for the labour ward kitchen.

'As you all know, I'm a very reasonable sister,' she said, which prompted nods of agreement from most of us gathered. 'I'm certainly not one to nit-pick about an extra pint of milk for your teas and coffees and the like. But if I don't get to the bottom of this I will have *Miss Sefton* asking questions, and we certainly don't want that, do we?'

An emphatic 'no' came from every person's lips.

'So please can somebody explain to me what is going on?'

Sister Penman knew that most of us midwives worked night shifts as well as days, and would no doubt be able to solve this great bicarbonate of soda mystery without the need for further intervention from Miss Sefton.

As the rest of us gave each other sideways glances, deciding who was going to spill the beans, one of the new pupil midwives bravely stepped forward.

'Sister Mallon makes pancakes for us on nights sometimes,' little Annie said, blushing. 'They're delicious, and we give them to the patients, too, if they want them. It's our fault, we're always asking her to make them.'

Sister Penman rolled her eyes. 'I honestly don't know how you find the time to be fiddle-faddling about with such things,' she chastised. 'Please don't encourage Sister Mallon any more. I have it on good authority that she's an impressive cook, but I think we must let her practise her skills at home from now on. I will have a word with her.'

We were all dismissed forthwith, stifling laughter as we thought about how our eyes twinkled when the overnight order sheet arrived and we all looked down the list and said, 'Oooh, let's have some of that!' or 'What shall we make next?'

It wasn't just kitchen supplies that we used a little lavishly. Since the move to the new unit and the shift to disposable equipment over the last few years, most of the staff had got into the habit of being really quite wasteful. It was such a revelation to us to have boxes of pre-sterilised needles and razors on hand, not to mention paper hats and plastic aprons, that we took full advantage. Even the bedpans were disposable now, made of a rigid grey card that could be dumped in a 'bedpan masher' – complete with their contents, thank goodness. Needless to say, nobody missed the old days of having to empty out the metal pans and wash them in the steriliser.

We were quite oblivious to the effect all the extra waste might have on the environment, and when it came to the plastics, recycling was not a word we were familiar with. Greenpeace was a fledgling organisation at this time, and I was vaguely aware of its anti-nuclear protests in Vancouver in the early Seventies, but to be honest I didn't make any connection between polluting the world with nuclear bombs and creating piles of NHS waste. I don't think I was alone in this ignorance, either. Midwives generally enjoyed the luxury of it all, knowing that the next box of shiny new supplies was only a tick on an order slip away, and rejoicing in the fact we no longer had to endure the smell of washing out metal bedpans.

If we ever did think twice about our actions, the extreme busyness of the wards gave us a good excuse for being profligate. On a typical day shift we had up to fifteen ladies arriving on the labour ward, and usually on nights five midwives would deliver two or three babies each, making us very grateful indeed to have such plentiful supplies so readily available.

On one such hectic shift, on a warm day in July 1973, I was dispatched to look after a new arrival on the labour ward. My patient was a rotund, jolly-looking lady called Rosemary Battersby. I will never forget her for many reasons, and she was actually the very first patient I confided in about my own pregnancy.

Examining Rosemary in the admissions room, I was surprised to see her labour was so well established that she really should have gone straight into a delivery room, but at that time there was a strict process we midwives were instructed to follow. All new arrivals were seen first in the admissions room, where many were still shaved and given an enema, provided labour was indeed established and they were already at least three centimetres dilated. Next, the women were taken to a first-stage room, where they laboured until they reached about nine to ten centimetres. Finally, when they were very nearly ready to push the baby out, they went into a delivery room.

Looking back it wasn't a good system, as it meant we were often shifting ladies between rooms when they were in the advanced stages of labour and could barely walk, let alone get on and off trolleys and beds. It was certainly not unusual to see women actually pushing as they were wheeled along corridors.

'My goodness, you've done a remarkable job all by yourself,' I said to Rosemary, seeing that she was already an impressive nine centimetres dilated.

'To be honest, I tried to put off comin' in until after the tennis,' she told me.

I knew Wimbledon was on, and there had been great excitement as it was the first time the women's final had been between two Americans, Billie Jean King and Chris Evert. I'm not a big tennis fan, though, and I hadn't really been following it.

'Well, I'm glad you're here now,' I told her.

When I felt Rosemary's huge abdomen, her contractions were frequent and strong, though she didn't appear to be suffering too much and even managed to give me a wide smile. I told her I was going to by-pass the first-stage room and take her straight to a delivery room as her labour was advancing so well, and I remarked that she appeared very good at dealing with the pain.

'I used to be a dancer,' she said proudly. 'Did the summer season at Blackpool for eight years running. My Billy reckons I must still have muscles of steel, under all this blubber!'

She let out a raucous laugh as she patted her tummy, and I laughed, too. This was her first baby, and I had a feeling I was going to really enjoy this birth.

'That's 'im there,' she said, nodding down the corridor as I helped her waddle carefully into a delivery room.

Billy was sitting on a plastic chair, his nose buried in a *Manchester Evening News*. ''Ere, Billy, wish me luck!' Rosemary called over, making him bounce up as if his seat had turned into a trampoline. He was a well-padded man with ruddy cheeks, a small goatee beard and long, straggly hair. I noticed he was wearing a purple jacket and wide-collared chocolate brown shirt, which made him look somewhat bohemian compared with most men I was used to seeing in Ashton.

Billy bounded up to us, looking a tad unbalanced in a pair of camel brown platform boots, and asked animatedly whether it was 'show time'.

'Nearly!' Rosemary chuckled. 'Midwife here says I'm ready to go straight into the labour room!'

Billy planted a noisy kiss on his wife's forehead and told her, 'Break a leg now, Rosie!'

'Is your husband in the entertainment business, too?' I asked once we'd got Rosemary into a hospital gown and she was lying down fairly comfortably, a foetal heart monitor strapped across her expansive belly.

'Oh yes,' she nodded.

Rosemary was huffing and puffing now, the effort of heaving herself onto the delivery bed seemingly giving her more grief than the labour pains themselves. Nevertheless, she was determined to tell me all about her Billy.

'He was a Redcoat at Butlins at Skegness before I knew him,' she panted. 'And we met when he joined a band and – uuuurggghhhh, that were a nasty one – did the summer season at Blackpoooowl. Ow, owww, owwwww! Is it meant to be hurting so much? I were fine a minute ago. He plays the ukulele like a dream.'

With that she let out a few rather musical notes of her own as the strength of her contractions intensified again and again, and yet again.

'I must be mad! Why am I doing this?' she wailed flamboyantly at one point, but I could tell she was simply letting off steam and was actually coping really well. Rosemary was clearly very comfortable taking centre stage, and even at the peak of labour she couldn't help holding forth.

'You ... urgh – you got any yerself, Nurse?' she asked me at one point, quite unexpectedly. 'Babies, I mean?'

'No ... but I'm just over three months pregnant!' I blurted out, astonishing myself momentarily with my revelation.

Rosemary's face lit up, and I felt a real connection to her.

'Good luck, nuuuurrgghhhhsseee! Sorry – sorry – sorry – I want to pu-pu-puuusssshhhhhh!'

It was less than fifteen minutes since we'd got her into this room, and no more than an hour since her arrival at the hospital, but I could see Rosemary was ready.

'OK, OK,' I said. 'Wait until I tell you, wait a bit, wait a bit, big breath – go now!'

Rosemary gave a substantial push and I could see the baby's head, advancing, just as I wanted it to.

'All right?' she puffed as she gasped for air.

'Brilliant,' I said. 'Magnificent!'

I wanted this wonderful performance to conclude well. Rosemary's sunny disposition had rubbed off on me, and I was enjoying this birth a great deal.

'I need the same again, when I tell you … OK, OK, go again, keep going …!'

An almighty cry filled the entire room moments later, heralding the arrival of a very rosy-faced, bright-eyed baby girl who landed with a little bump on the bed. Scooping her up, my eyes immediately fell on the baby's left arm. Instinctively, I reached for a cotton towel and draped it over the baby, leaving only her pretty little face peeping out.

I was very upset by what I'd seen. At the end of the baby's left arm there was no hand. It was just a little stump, with a tiny bud of a thumb and no fingers. Rosemary was propped up on her elbows now, her eyes darting between her large deflated stomach and the baby in my arms. She seemed stunned into silence by the speed of the delivery, which had left her dragging in breath noisily. She could not have seen her daughter's arm; I had covered her up so quickly I was sure Rosemary hadn't seen what I had. It was down to me to break the news.

'Congratulations Rosemary,' I smiled warmly. 'You have a lovely baby daughter.'

I remembered hearing of a scenario like this during my training, when I was out in the community with Mrs Tattersall. She had told me how one of her colleagues delivered a breech baby who had a deformed foot. It was a difficult situation because the baby's legs were delivered first and so the community midwife knew many minutes before the baby was even born that there was a problem. I fast-forwarded in my mind to what Mrs Tattersall's answer had been when I asked her how you should deal with such a case.

'Let mum see the baby and look at the baby,' I heard Mrs Tattersall's raspy voice say. 'If she doesn't remark on the deformity herself, you need to refer to it gently, in a very nice manner, of course. "Unfortunately, your baby's foot is a little deformed," you should say. "But there are things you and he can use to help, and I'm sure he will cope well …"'

I cut the cord and delivered the placenta as Rosemary lay back, quiet with exhaustion. 'Is she all right?' she asked softly. 'Can I see her?'

The baby was wrapped snugly in a blanket now. I lifted her over, letting Rosemary feast her eyes on her daughter's beautiful face for a moment before I loosened the cover. The little girl cried when the air hit her bare chest. Her legs wriggled and she shot both arms up in a reflex action, just as a newborn should.

Rosemary's eyes fell on her daughter's arm, and I was very comforted by the fact I could still hear Mrs Tattersall guiding me.

'Wh-wh-what's happened to her hand?' Rosemary asked slowly. 'Is it my ff-fault?' Tears were welling in her eyes. 'W-w-what did I do wrong?'

'You did absolutely nothing wrong at all,' I replied, handing her the snuffling baby to cuddle. 'It is just one of those things. I'm sure you must know other children who were born with little things not quite right. It happens, but I'm sure she'll cope really well.'

'Poor little soul,' Rosemary said, giving the little girl a gentle kiss on the forehead.

I swear Mrs Tattersall dug her bony elbow into my rib at that precise moment, prompting me to add, 'If you look, she's got this little bud here in place of a thumb, which is good. It will help her to grip things.' The words came out of my mouth, but they had been planted firmly in my head by Mrs Tattersall, and I silently thanked her.

When Rosemary indicated she was ready to see her husband, I asked Billy to step inside and meet his new baby daughter. I could see they were a solid, close couple and I would let Rosemary tell him the news in her own way and in her own good time. I would stay close by, busying myself with writing up the notes and tidying up, so as not to intrude but to be there if they needed me.

What happened next was incredibly heart-warming. Unbeknown to me, Billy had brought his ukulele into the maternity unit. It seemed he had planned all along to serenade his wife and new child, and this unfortunate turn of events had not dented his enthusiasm.

'I would have waited a bit, you know, if things …' he explained to me as he took the instrument slowly from its case. 'But … can I?'

I nodded and made sure the door was shut behind us, and then I watched and listened, spellbound, as Billy gently strummed his ukulele and gave a brief rendition of 'All You Need is Love.'

Rosemary rocked the baby in her arms and sobbed quietly before saying, 'Come 'ere, ya soppy old devil!'

Billy put his arms around both his wife and new baby daughter, and I knew in that moment that what Mrs Tattersall had said to me many times was so true. 'People cope, you'd be surprised Linda. There are always ways around things. It usually works out in the end.' These were all typical Mrs Tattersall sayings, and how very right she was.

When I went home that night, I didn't tell Graham a thing. I didn't want him to start worrying about our own baby, and I didn't feel the need to unload on him. I actually felt surprisingly at ease about the events of the day, and when I jotted down a few thoughts and feelings in my notebook, as I sometimes did, I realised why.

'People keep asking me if being a midwife hasn't put me off having babies of my own,' I wrote as I sat on our bed at home. 'I think it has the opposite effect. I can't wait to have my baby! If being a midwife has taught me anything, it is that, come what may, babies bring a great deal of happiness.'

'Billy Jean King beat Chris Evert 6–0, 7–5. Did you hear?' Graham called up the stairs to me.

'No, missed that,' I replied. 'Been a bit busy today.'

'Not too busy, I hope?' Graham asked protectively. 'Not in your condition!'

I loved that he was looking out for me, but I reassured him that I was absolutely fine, and that I was perfectly capable of working through my pregnancy, especially at this early stage as I was still only just into my fourth month. Despite the trials of the day I knew I had done a good job and I felt sure Rosemary and Billy's baby would thrive, having such inspiring parents.

Graham and I would be good parents, too, I knew it. We loved each other very much, and as Billy had made clear so very touchingly, love really is all you need.

Chapter Four

'I think I've eaten far too much turkey'

My pregnancy was progressing well. It was October 1973 and I was six months pregnant and feeling absolutely wonderful. Save for the fact I'd been issued with bigger uniforms that accommodated my growing bump but gaped unflatteringly around my bust, you would hardly have known I was pregnant. I had no morning sickness, never had any problems at my antenatal appointments and I felt fit and well. In fact, I felt so good that I decided to work right up until thirty-six weeks, even though I was entitled to stop at twenty-nine weeks, which was what the majority of women did at that time.

Graham and I had just moved into a semi-detached house on Four Lanes in Mottram. It cost £9,999 and was another step up the ladder for us. I loved my kitchen. It had a fashionable peninsular unit, small flowers inlaid into the design of the worktop and fluorescent lights, which were very trendy. On the worktop I even had an electric cake mixer, which was considered to be a very posh gadget at that time. We also had a central heating system fitted in the ceiling, no less, which was very modern (though not very efficient); we decorated every wall with the latest woodchip paper and, most important of all, we decided to splash out on brand new teak G-plan furniture.

'Oh, you're really somebody when you've got G-plan furniture!' my brother John joked when he telephoned from his home in Vienna one night.

He was teasing, of course, but what he said actually rang true. We felt we'd really arrived, Graham and I, at least in our little corner of Ashton-under-Lyne.

My brother was still working very successfully as a journalist, and his wife Nevim was busy being a mum and learning French. Little Kerem was two years old by now and baby Tijen was five months old. We didn't see a great deal of the family, as travel was expensive back then, but we always tried to keep in touch on the telephone and I'd always look forward to their occasional visits at Christmas.

I knew that our parents were very proud of the way John and I had turned out. With such a big age gap between us I had never really seen myself as an equal to John, not until now. The fact he was a full ten years older than me meant I had always looked up to him, but as I was about to become a parent myself, and I was now twenty-five years old, I no longer felt like the much younger little sister I always had been. I was as secure and settled and grown-up as him, and it was a good feeling to acknowledge.

Together, Graham and I turned one of our three bedrooms into a nursery in preparation for the baby, installing a beautiful white cot and a matching wardrobe and chest of drawers.

'I don't want you overdoing things,' Graham said when I insisted on going up the ladder to help paint white emulsion over the woodchip, before adding an animal design frieze.

'I'm fine!' I said. 'You know me, I like to be busy.'

'That's what bothers me. Are you *sure* they're looking after you at work?'

'Of course they are. I could hardly be in a better place, could I?'

My colleagues often encouraged me to put my feet up in the day room for half an hour if it were possible, and I told Graham that I was coping really well and really enjoying working through my pregnancy. It was true. Nothing could have been better. I was in a good phase of my life, in every sense.

One lunchtime around this time, a beautiful young Asian woman arrived on the labour ward. There was a very small Asian population in Ashton in those days, and the few Asian women we did see at the hospital spoke hardly any English. There was usually another cultural barrier to overcome, too, as the Asian ladies we encountered were usually extremely modest and did not like to remove their clothing or have any men in the room during examinations or deliveries, consultants included. If there were any potential complications, sometimes the midwives tried to get a female doctor on standby, as there were no female consultants back then.

This particular lady, who according to her notes was happy to be addressed by her first name, Sangheeta, arrived with a slightly older woman who I assumed to be her sister, as they looked very much alike.

'I would like to examine you,' I said, showing Sangheeta onto a bed in an admissions room. 'Is it possible to lift your clothing?' I raised the bottom of my apron to demonstrate what I meant.

Sangheeta lowered her eyes and batted her long eyelashes bashfully while her sister shook her head. 'You feel,' the sister instructed, gesturing for me to put my hands on Sangheeta's abdomen, on top of her clothing.

I didn't want to offend the sisters in any way at this very early stage. Only a few weeks earlier, we'd had an awkward incident on the ward with one of our long-serving midwives, Erica, who was Nigerian. A patient had given her a box of Black Magic chocolates as a thank-you gift, which Erica had taken as a dig, although it was meant as nothing of the sort.

'Take those away!' she had shouted. 'Does she think this is funny? Get them out of my sight!'

Her reaction had shocked me as well as several colleagues who also witnessed Erica's outburst. The vast majority of the midwives were white, but we were most certainly not racist in any way. Erica was being unnecessarily paranoid, even though, looking back, I can see how it might have been a bit tough for her to be in such a very small minority.

I didn't want to create any unnecessary tension with Sangheeta and so I assessed her face to see how she was coping, as facial expressions are often a good indicator of how a patient is managing the pain. She was not grimacing and appeared to be at ease – serene, even – as I got her to lie back on the bed so I could put my hand over her clothing to feel the strength of the contractions.

Her abdomen felt tight but the contractions were not strong at all, and were very few and far between. According to her notes this was her first baby, which meant it was not likely to come quickly. I decided it was perfectly safe to leave her under the watchful eye of her sister for a little while, as I had several other jobs to do.

'Can you deal with Mrs Cox?' Sister Penman asked urgently a few minutes later. I had hoped to grab a quick word with a lady I'd delivered earlier that day but, by the sound of it, Mrs Cox would have to come first.

'She's in the first-stage room, giving her husband a terribly hard time, I'm afraid. I've only got a pupil midwife free otherwise, and I'd rather you took this one.'

'No problem,' I said. 'I'll be right there.'

Before I entered the first-stage room, I poked my head quickly back round the door of the admissions room and was pleased to see Sangheeta lying back as serenely as before, a sheet now pulled up protectively over her clothes.

'I'll be back as soon as I can,' I said, to which Sangheeta and her sister smiled politely, if blankly.

Crossing the corridor, I heard Mrs Cox before I saw her and I stopped in my tracks.

'Effing hell,' she shrieked loudly. 'Christ Almighty! Get your effing hands off me you effing lunatic!'

I was used to hearing women swearing and shouting during labour – or effing and jeffing, as I call it – but Mrs Cox sounded more hysterical and aggressive than any women I had ever encountered. I took a deep breath and entered the room.

I was shocked to see that Mrs Cox was lashing out at her husband, kicking and hitting and scratching him quite violently as he tried to hold her down on the bed. Her eyes were wild with anxiety.

'Don't you effing dare! Eff off! You effing, effing – bastard!!'

Mr Cox looked pale and visibly shaken as he struggled to restrain his wife.

'Thank God you're here, Nurse,' he said in a trembling voice. 'I don't know what to do. She kicked off on the ambulancemen, too, they had a job getting her in here. It's so unlike her. I've never seen her like this before!'

I actually recognised Mrs Cox, though I didn't know her. She worked behind the counter of one of the shops on the parade near our house, and she was usually the most polite and mild-mannered woman you could wish to meet.

'Sometimes this can happen,' I explained to Mr Cox. 'Women cope with the pains of labour in so many different ways, and sometimes a woman's personality changes completely when she's in labour.'

'What do you effing know about it you effing BITCH!' Mrs Cox hollered. 'Effing midwives think they effing know it all!'

Mr Cox looked absolutely mortified and apologised profusely.

'I see you're pregnant yourself, Nurse,' he said. 'I'm terribly sorry about this. How many have you got?'

When I told him this was my first baby, Mrs Cox let rip again, pointing at me accusingly and telling me I didn't have an 'effing clue' what I was talking about. It was clear that soothing words from me were not going to calm Mrs Cox; she was far too distressed for that.

'Mrs Cox!' I said, raising my voice sternly. 'I am *very* offended by your language and I don't want any more of it, do you hear me? Please stop swearing *right now*!'

She grunted rudely at me, but thankfully my words shook her into silence long enough for me to administer some pain relief while Mr Cox held her down as steady as he could for me. I gave her an injection of Pethidine and, much to my relief, when the drug took hold Mrs Cox stopped thrashing and kicking and lay very still between her mild contractions, albeit with eyes still blazing and with a terrible scowl carved on her face.

'I truly can't apologise enough,' Mr Cox said, shaking his head from side to side.

'Honestly, don't worry,' I replied. 'Just please stay right with her. Even though she is calmer now, I don't want you to leave the bedside in case she starts up again. I need to slip out for a moment, but I'll be right back.'

I dashed across the corridor to check on Sangheeta, figuring I would get the pupil midwife to take over her care as soon as it was necessary. It was not uncommon for me to be looking after two ladies at the same time, particularly when they were both in the early stages of labour, as both Sangheeta and Mrs Cox were, but on this occasion I wanted to focus fully on Mrs Cox.

Sangheeta's sister was coming out of the admissions room just as I arrived at the door, and she pulled my arm, urging me into the room. She looked a little flustered and as I stepped inside the room I was relieved to see Sangheeta was still lying calmly on the bed, now with her knees up but still covered by the sheet.

'I would really like to have a closer look at you now,' I said, at which point Sangheeta's sister stepped forward silently, and gently lifted the sheet.

I gasped in surprise. There, blinking up at me from between Sangheeta's legs, was a very pretty little baby girl. She had the most beautiful long eyelashes, just like her mum, and was absolutely captivating. Mother and daughter were clearly no worse for wear for not having had a midwife at the birth, and I smiled at Sangheeta and said, 'Clever girl'. She smiled sweetly back at me and I knew she understood.

Looking around the room, I saw a clean towel and indicated to Sangheeta that I wanted to wrap the baby in it. I rang the bell and, when help arrived, I gave Sangheeta an injection of Syntometrine and cut the baby's umbilical cord. Once the third stage was complete and all was well, I asked the pupil midwife to take over from me, allowing me to return to the lion's den, or at least the delivery room that Mrs Cox was labouring in.

It was several extremely long hours before Mrs Cox reached the second stage and was ready to push, and I honestly don't know who was more exhausted – me, her or her husband! She had continued to swear and curse on and off throughout the labour, though thankfully her hitting and kicking subsided towards the end, even when her pain relief wore off, no doubt because she couldn't possibly have had the energy to keep it up for so many hours.

When it was time to deliver the baby, however, Mrs Cox began to thrash very violently again. She began lashing out like a mad woman, in fact, effing and grunting and whacking her poor husband repeatedly as she pushed the baby out.

'Hang on to her tight,' I instructed Mr Cox. 'We can't have her falling off the bed.'

When the baby's head emerged, I actually had a job holding on to it as Mrs Cox was writhing around so forcefully, jolting her body from side to side as if she were being electrocuted. Several pushes and dozens more expletives later, baby Cox landed on the bed and let out a wail that was very loud, but nowhere near as deafening as one of her mother's.

'It's a girl!' I announced breathlessly. 'Well done!' My arms and hands were shaking as I lifted the baby up.

'Thank you,' Mrs Cox whimpered, slumping onto her pillow with exhaustion. 'I'm so, so, sorry. So sorry, really I am.'

'It's fine,' I smiled.

Mrs Cox watched me silently through her tired eyes as I cut the cord, and she then went on to deliver the placenta incredibly placidly.

'Isn't she just so beautiful,' she cooed, gazing at her dainty baby girl.

It was as if a switch had been thrown in Mrs Cox's brain. Her voice was angelic, her manner so peaceful. You could have heard a pin drop as I cleaned the blood off the baby's head, weighed her in at exactly seven pounds and placed her in a nappy and a nightie before letting Mrs Cox have her first hold.

'I knew a woman could get a bit agitated in labour, but I didn't expect my wife to have a complete personality transplant,' Mr Cox said several hours later, when I visited the new family on the postnatal ward at the end of my shift.

'Once again, Nurse, I can't apologise enough. I'm so, so sorry,' Mrs Cox repeated.

Her voice was croaky and she was sucking on an Uncle Joe's Mint Balls boiled sweet to soothe her hoarse throat. She was deeply embarrassed and told me she didn't know what had come over her. Mr Cox had bruises and scratches all up his arms, and he saw me notice them.

'Next time, I'm going to make sure she cuts her nails,' he joked, at which point Mrs Cox gave him a playful shove.

'Next time?' she said. 'Are you kidding me? I'm never going through that again!'

I left them to it and went home, thinking to myself that I was sure there *would* be a next time, despite what the couple had been through and what they were saying now. Nature has a way of making women forget, and I was sure Mrs Cox would be back again one day, probably in the not-too-distant future and no doubt kicking and screaming and hurting her throat once more as she provided a sibling for little Grace, as they named the baby. Yes, the name tickled me no end, after the far from graceful scenes we'd had in the delivery room!

'Another busy day?' Graham asked as I set about grilling some chops for tea that night.

'So-so,' I replied, not wanting him to fuss over me, even though on this occasion I felt both physically and mentally worn out.

'How many did you deliver today?'

'Oh, just two,' I replied honestly, thinking I couldn't claim to have delivered Sangheeta's baby.

'That's good, a quiet day for you, then. Glad to hear it, my little midwife.'

I went upstairs to change out of my uniform and into some maternity clothes, choosing a comfortable smock dress over a floral blouse with a Peter Pan collar. In those days we tried to hide our bumps, not show them off, and so I lived in either smocks or pinafore dresses when I wasn't at work.

As I dressed I smiled to myself, imagining what an eye-opener it would be for Graham when he came into hospital to see our baby being born. I had already decided I wanted him to witness the birth and he had readily agreed, saying that if I wanted him there he trusted it was the best thing to do. I'd seen how bonding it could be for couples to share the experience, and I also wanted Graham with me for moral support. I couldn't imagine not having him there, actually. I could have chosen a home birth, as I had no complications, but I instinctively wanted to be in the hospital, with Graham at my side. It just felt right for me.

I went into the kitchen and washed a handful of potatoes, peeled them and set them to boil on the hob. The whole business of preparing the meal was so much more labour-intensive back then. Potatoes and vegetables bought on Ashton market were always caked in soil. There was no such thing as picking up a bag of pre-cut carrots in the supermarket, or simply putting a neat sachet of vegetables in the microwave to steam for two minutes. I always made gravy from scratch using Bisto powder, as there were no instant granules, and if we wanted apple sauce with our chops I'd stew a cooking apple and make my own. Then, after the meal, there would always be a stack of washing-up to tackle because of course we didn't have a dishwasher.

As I grilled the chops that evening I amused myself by picturing Graham's face when he saw midwives dashing around the corridors, attending to three, four or even five labouring women at a time, which would no doubt be the scenario when I went in to have my baby.

'This is a quiet day,' I would tell him, and enjoy watching his jaw hit the floor in surprise.

In early December 1973 I started my maternity leave, as my due date of 7 January 1974 was just four weeks away. It was a treat to have most of the month off so I could put the finishing touches to the nursery, relax a bit and enjoy the festive season. My mum took me shopping in Macclesfield and bought me a beautiful navy-and-cream Marmet pram that bounced along on a huge chassis, like something out of *Mary Poppins*, and my in-laws paid for the new cot in the nursery and also gave us a lovely carrycot. Graham splashed out, too, buying me a white Mini convertible van so I could fit the large pram into the back, while friends and relatives were all busy knitting cot blankets, cardigans, bootees and mittens.

On several occasions I took myself off to The Beehive, a smart children's boutique in Stalybridge, where I enjoyed picking out babygros and bibs and little socks. Everything I bought was either white, cream or yellow. Without the benefit of ultrasound scans, which were many years away yet, we had no clue as to whether I was expecting a boy or a girl. That was about the only unknown, however. Everything else was as neatly arranged and organised as could be. We couldn't have been better prepared, I thought, and I looked forward to Christmas and the New Year very much.

My mum insisted on buying us a turkey and went completely over the top. I think it weighed about eighteen pounds despite there being only my parents, Graham and me for Christmas dinner at our house. As a result we found ourselves eating turkey sandwiches, turkey soup and yet more turkey sandwiches for days afterwards.

'I think I've eaten far too much turkey,' I grumbled to Graham as we headed up to bed at 10.30 p.m. on 28 December. 'I've got terrible indigestion.'

'Can I get you anything?'

'No, you go to sleep. It'll probably settle when I lie down.'

My stomach pains were so bad, however, that I hardly slept at all, and at 6 a.m. I went downstairs and started pacing around the settee, clutching my bump. It was only after about ten minutes that the penny dropped, and I realised I was not suffering from indigestion at all: I was in the first stage of labour. I felt such a fool, not realising this straightaway, but in my mind this baby was arriving on 7 January, as planned.

I paced around the lounge for more than an hour on my own, breathing through my contractions and coping well with the pain. I didn't wake Graham until about 7.30, not wanting him to lose sleep unnecessarily.

'I think we'd better get up to the hospital soon,' I blurted. 'The baby's coming early!'

We arrived on the labour ward at 8.30 and I was really pleased and relieved to see that Judith Houghton was on duty and would be able to deliver me. There was something very comforting about this, with Judith having guided my hands the very first time I delivered a baby. She was an extremely experienced midwife and I knew I would in very capable hands, which was just as well as I was beginning to buckle under the pain.

'I can't do this!' I told Judith as she got me on a bed in the first-stage room and examined me.

'Of course you can, Linda,' she soothed. 'Let's have a look … Oh, my goodness, you have done ever so well, without any pain relief. You're seven centimetres already!'

It certainly wasn't uncommon for women to leave it this late to come into hospital, but usually that was because they didn't have any experience of labour and did not realise how close to delivering their baby they were. It might have been better if I'd gone in earlier, but I just hadn't realised how far I'd got on my own, despite my job. By this point, though, I was in too much pain to bother about what anybody thought of me. I was just so glad I was well established in labour, and that this was not a false alarm.

'Can I have some Pethidine, please?'

'Of course,' Judith responded. 'You'll have some pain relief any minute now, Linda.'

I'd avoided a shave and enema, thank goodness. This was not special treatment. They were no longer routinely given, and in my case my labour was progressing so quickly there really wasn't time, though I'm sure Judith would have let me off in any case.

As I was swiftly transferred into a delivery room I cursed the system that meant I had to get off one bed, onto a trolley and then struggle from the trolley onto the delivery bed in my cumbersome condition. No wonder my ladies always complained about this; it was ridiculously inconvenient. I began to sob as a huge contraction rippled across my abdomen. This was absolute agony, and I wanted it all to end, right this very second.

'Aaarrrgghh!' I shrieked, clutching Graham's hand so hard I felt his bones click. 'I can't do it! I can't do it. Where's the Pethidine? Give me the PETHIDINE!!'

I saw that Graham's face was filled with worry and bemusement. In all our years together he had rarely seen me raise my voice before, let alone behave like this. I'd told him plenty of stories of how other women carried on when they gave birth, but I think he thought that only happened to other people, and certainly not to a mild-mannered midwife like me.

Graham was very much mistaken, though, and I must admit I shocked myself, too. I was acting exactly like plenty of women I had delivered, many of whom I had told to quieten down or had felt embarrassed for when the pain had made them lose control, just as I was doing.

'I want my mum!' I bellowed when Judith explained that she was going to perform an episiotomy, to reduce the chances of tearing. 'I know what an episiotomy is! Where's my mum? I can't do this any more.'

It did not come as any surprise that I was having an episiotomy, as most women still had one in those days rather than risking a tear, which was considered quite a disgrace by midwives. However, knowing the theory was about to become a reality set me off shouting even louder.

'I want my mum and I want to go home NOOOOWWWW!' I screeched, clamping my hand around Graham's arm and staring frantically at the ceiling, my head clamped to the pillow as I gritted my teeth between shouts.

Jonathan was born at 10.40 a.m. and weighed eight pounds, three ounces. He cried straightaway, and when Judith handed him to me, wrapped in a blanket, I fell in love with him right there and then. He had sandy-coloured hair and a little squashed face; he was a big, chunky baby for me and it must have been a tight squeeze for him.

When I looked at him I was the only woman in the world who had a baby, and the only woman in the world who loved her baby as much as I loved Jonathan. That's how I felt, lying in this room that was normally my workplace, marvelling at this new life, this tiny person, who was now such a huge responsibility to me. It was absolutely mind-blowing.

Graham was besotted, too. 'Well done, love,' he said, kissing my hot forehead, which was drenched in sweat. He couldn't take his eyes off Jonathan. He was absolutely thrilled to bits, not to mention rather relieved to see me behaving in my normal, calm manner again.

'I hardly recognised you for a while there, Linda,' he said, exhaling slowly, still looking slightly shell-shocked.

I caught a glimpse of Judith smiling to herself as she wrote up my notes. No doubt she was recalling our conversation of a few months earlier, when I'd rather naïvely promised to be a model patient. How could I have thought I wouldn't create a fuss like so many other women? I was exactly like them, midwife or not, and I was so glad I was. I was a mum now, and I had joined the most special club in the world.

I remember my postnatal stay in hospital vividly. Even though breastfeeding was still not very popular back then, I wanted to give it a go, having learned the benefits of breastmilk through my training. It was also expected of midwives to set a good example. I was given a side room all to myself so I could learn how to feed quietly, but as soon as I was able I went to the day room to meet some other mums. There I talked to a friendly lady called Sybil who had given birth on the same day as me to her son Robert. Sybil told me that the other patients were quite animated about the fact one of the hospital's own midwives – and a sister, no less! – was on the same ward as them, albeit in the side room.

It was very easy to chat to Sybil. There is something very bonding about having been through such a dramatic experience as childbirth at the very same time, and I felt like I'd known her for ages. I'd seen instant friendships like mine and Sybil's formed countless times when I was working on the postnatal ward, and it was always heartening to watch the new mothers getting along and supporting each other so effortlessly whilst in hospital.

Sybil and I didn't keep in regular touch when we both eventually left hospital the following week, but I never forgot her. To this day we still bump into each other occasionally when out shopping in Glossop, and we never fail to talk about Jonathan and Robert, and how they are both getting along.

During my time in hospital I also recall being bowled over by the generosity of my colleagues, who presented me with a gigantic box crammed full of all sorts of goodies like baby creams, cotton wool, shampoo and newborn baby clothes that they had all clubbed together to buy.

Those were the high points of my stay, but mostly I have to admit I remember feeling absolutely, totally and utterly exhausted. I seemed to have a non-stop stream of visitors. Every one of my midwife friends popped in to see me. Every relative, every friend, every neighbour came to have a peep at Jonathan. Graham was given a bit more leniency than other dads when it came to visiting hours, and so he was nipping in and out all the time, too. I smiled, I was ever so polite and I let everyone have a hold of my precious baby, but by the third day I was desperately wishing for some peace and quiet, and some time alone to get to know my gorgeous but very demanding little boy.

'Will I fetch yer a hot orange?' Sister Kelly offered when she came to see me.

It seemed quite surreal to be sitting there in my Marks and Spencer nightdress and new fluffy white dressing gown while my colleagues were all in uniform, and talking to me just the same as they always did.

'No thanks,' I replied, thinking I would have preferred her to offer to limit the flow of visitors or to change Jonathan's nappy than to bring me hot orange.

I actually felt quite tearful, in fact. None of the sisters, midwives or auxiliaries on the ward wanted to be seen to be interfering with anything I was doing, which meant I didn't get the same help the other new mums received when it came to changing, feeding and bathing my baby. I was a competent, experienced midwife; I was not in need of any assistance what-soever with my son. That's what everybody thought, and I certainly didn't want to disappoint them, so I tried to be perfect, all on my own, despite being a complete beginner when it came to being a mother.

Sister Kelly encouraged me to stay in hospital for as long as possible. 'Get yerself rested, get the breastfeeding established while you've not got to think about cookin' an' cleanin' at home, Linda,' she said kindly. 'Enjoy the break!'

All of my colleagues were trying to be so kind and helpful, constantly checking up on me and nipping in for a chat and a cuddle of the baby, but in the end I was desperate to get out of hospital because I was absolutely worn out. Jonathan was eight days old when I finally took him home.

'I can't tell you how good it is to sleep in my own bed,' I told Graham that night.

'I can't tell you how good it is to have you back,' he replied.

I expected everything to be wonderful from that moment on, but unfortunately it wasn't. I really struggled to feed Jonathan and it was challenging trying to keep the house as spick and span as I liked it, while also dealing with new chores like soaking nappies in a bucket before washing them, and getting up two, three or even four times during the night.

'Can I help?' Graham said many times. 'No, no, I'm fine,' I always replied.

It wasn't the done thing for men to get involved in changing nappies or washing baby clothes in those days, and so I did everything, willingly. I wasn't complaining, because I loved Jonathan so much despite finding it hard to adjust to the demands of motherhood. Just holding him gave me a wonderful warm glow, and when I looked into his eyes I felt besotted and devoted to him. It reminded me of the feeling of joy I felt each time I brought a baby into the world – except, of course, with Jonathan I didn't hand him over to another woman afterwards and then go about my normal business.

Jonathan was an all-consuming, full-time job, and the hardest job I had ever done. I was struggling, though I couldn't admit this to anyone. Whenever Mum came round to help me out I made polite conversation and smiled. I'd tell her, 'Just leave it to me,' whenever she offered to wash out the nappies or iron Graham's shirts. 'I can do it all, it's not as if I'm working.'

My father just played the jovial grandfather, as men did in those days. I never recall talking about emotions or how I really felt with either my mother or my father, but I think that was quite typical of the day. My parents had brought me up well. I had a good job, a lovely home and a suitable husband. Now I'd produced a beautiful grandchild for them, too. My life was complete. How could I even think about saying I was finding it a bit tough bringing up a baby?

I had one or two postnatal visits from colleagues, which was far fewer than other women received. I nodded in agreement when they said things like, 'Seems daft visiting you, Linda. If you don't know what's what then I don't know who does!'

It therefore came as a huge shock to everyone when my mum found me staggering about one evening with a vacant look in my eyes and in obvious pain. I was on the landing, with three-week old Jonathan in my arms. I have very little recollection of what was happening to me, but Mum said I began to sob and she couldn't get any sense out me. It seems I was delirious through lack of sleep, and because of a searing, dreadful pain I was experiencing in my breasts.

I had not acknowledged the extent of this pain to anyone, perhaps even myself, until I reached this crisis point and could bear it no more. I do recall the pain seemed to spill out in all directions around my body, making my nerves jangle and my head pound, as if I had a horrible flu bug.

'I think we need to get the doctor to come and see you,' Mum said straightaway, and I didn't argue; in fact I cried with relief.

The next few hours are quite a fog in my mind, but I remember finding myself sitting up in bed on a surgical ward at Ashton General with a doctor I had never seen before peering down at me through half-moon spectacles.

'You have breast abscesses caused by mastitis,' he explained. 'As you have unfortunately found out, this is a very painful condition that breastfeeding mothers sometimes suffer from. It happens when the milk ducts get blocked, often because breastfeeding has stopped suddenly, and it can cause a high temperature and flu-like symptoms and a great deal of pain.'

Scanning my notes, he raised an eyebrow and added, 'I see you are a midwife here, so I trust you know all this already.'

I nodded uncertainly and acknowledged that I had struggled so much with breastfeeding that I had stopped suddenly overnight, practically as soon as I got home from hospital with Jonathan when he was eight days old. I thought I was doing the right thing, as Jonathan was a hungry baby and I wasn't providing enough milk for him. I had forgotten the golden rule, which is that you are meant to wean the baby off the breast slowly, and then I'd naïvely thought that the pain I experienced was simply a reaction to my stopping breastfeeding.

I felt quite foolish, but I'd never come across mastitis in my work. So few women breastfed and, besides, as a midwife it was simply my role to help and advise women to breastfeed while in hospital, in the first few days of the baby's life. I had not encountered such a complication either during my time out in the community with Mrs Tattersall as a pupil midwife, or on the postnatal wards in recent years.

The sympathetic doctor went on to explain that unfortunately I was in a very small minority of women whose mastitis went on to cause breast abscesses, probably as a result of the milk trapped in the breast becoming infected. I had developed abscesses in one breast, and would need a minor operation to drain them.

I cried forlornly, and when Graham visited me later I cried again.

'I'm so sorry,' I told him. 'I'm really sorry.' I felt such a failure.

'It's not your fault,' he said. 'Your mum and my mum are helping me with Jonathan. Don't worry, just get better.'

I think he said the same thing every single day for a week, each time he visited. It turned out I needed my other breast operating on, too, and I had two bottles tightly clamped to either side of my chest, into which the infection was drained. I remember sitting in the day room in my dressing gown, suffering dreadfully with the pain and feeling so wiped out I could barely turn the pages of a magazine or pass the time of day with other patients.

'I'm feeling better, thanks' I always told Graham, attempting a smile whenever he visited.

Inside, however, I felt very blue – depressed, even. Whenever someone brought Jonathan to the window for me to see it lifted my spirits no end, but when I was alone again I felt very low. He wasn't allowed onto the ward, as babies and children were kept out of general wards in the hospital, for fear of them catching an infection. I felt I had failed in a basic maternal task, and I didn't like it one bit. I thought I would make a super new mum, just as everybody told me I would, but I'd let them all down. I couldn't even do something as natural as breastfeeding, and now I couldn't even cuddle my son. It seemed like the end of the world.

I spent a lot of time wiping tears from my eyes, caused both by pain and sorrow. I'd never felt so terrible in my life before, and I was consumed with a pessimism I was very unused to. I desperately wanted to go home, but I was also worried about how I could cope alone, feeling as wretched as I did. I began to look at Graham with a little bit of resentment, if I'm honest. In sharp contrast to me, his body was unchanged and he still went to work as normal, as well as going out socialising with his brother or his friends. My life had been completely turned upside down, and it was hard to get my head around so many changes.

When I was finally discharged and was able to sleep in my own bed once more, the relief and comfort I'd imagined at home just wasn't there. I'd been in hospital for a week and was well on the road to a physical recovery, but I was still healing and feeling very sore. Having Graham lying next to me in bed was quite unbearable. Each time he moved or turned over my body rippled with pain. I couldn't stand it, and I had to ask him to sleep on the floor beside the bed. He didn't grumble, but the physical divide was clearly not healthy for our relationship. I didn't have the capacity to compute this fact at the time, however. All my attention was on trying to feel normal and well again, so I could start to fully enjoy my baby.

Looking back, I can see I suffered from a mild dose of postnatal depression, though in those days it did not have a name and was not really spoken about. 'Oh, she's got a bit of baby blues' was about as much as was said about such matters. As a midwife, I knew it was common for new mothers to be tearful, particularly on the third day after giving birth. This was recognised and accepted as a normal hormonal response to delivering a baby and starting to produce milk.

The ongoing mental and psychological reaction a mother might have to this seismic change in her life was not discussed, however. The magnitude of the impact of having a baby on your career, your marriage, your entire view on the world was many years away from being talked about openly over dinner tables or dissected on television programmes.

For a midwife in 1974 to hold up her hand and say she wasn't feeling anything other than wonderful now she was a mother herself was absolutely unheard of, and so I bravely kept the silence, month after month.

In October 1974 Graham and I took ten-month-old Jonathan with us on a week-long package holiday to Magaluf, which was quite something in those days as most of our friends still holidayed in the UK, especially those with young children.

'This is the life!' Graham declared as we went sightseeing and ate lovely meals in the hotel's smart restaurant.

Jonathan was as good as gold and slept soundly in an iron cot in our room. When we all went down to breakfast together or strolled along the promenade with Jonathan in his buggy, I felt good. I'd started to do a bit of sewing at home and I wore flared A-line skirts I'd made from fashionable tartan material, which I paired with pretty frilled summer blouses draped with strings of cheap glass beads. I had loads of sets of them, most bought on Ashton market, but I remember I added to my jewellery collection when we visited the local Andratx market, as beads like that were all the rage out there and only cost a few pesetas.

'Yes, this is the life,' I agreed with Graham, and I really meant it.

I couldn't put my finger on exactly when I'd emerged from the difficult early days of motherhood that had dragged me down, but on that holiday I certainly felt back to my old self, and it wasn't just because of the sun, sand and occasional glass of Sangria. I'd got back on track, and I felt happy and fulfilled.

'Are you looking forward to going back to work?' Dad asked when he came to collect us from Manchester Airport. It was a damp and cold afternoon, and grey drizzle was descending all around dad's car, but the sky felt clear above my head. To tell the truth, I was still buzzing from the flight, as air travel was very exciting in those days and even having a meal on the plane was really quite a thrilling treat. You were made to feel like a privileged customer, even in economy class, and I felt fantastic.

'Yes I am looking forward to it,' I beamed. 'I'm a bit nervous too, but I can't wait. How's Mum?'

'Very well,' Dad said. 'There's no news. You haven't missed anything.'

Mum still did her little part-time job at the hospital and I'd been quite envious of her some days during my maternity leave, seeing how animated she became when she talked about the characters she'd met, or repeated a funny story she'd heard on her break. I never confided in her about just how awful I'd felt in the first few months of Jonathan's life. None of my close friends or family really questioned me about what it was like to have become so ill, and I didn't volunteer any information. I was glad now, because it was all in the past. I was more than ready to go back to work. It meant I could click back into being Linda, the capable midwife. It was a role I always felt completely comfortable in.

Chapter Five

'Help me! I'm boiling me 'ead off!'

I took a deep breath as I reported for duty for the first time in eleven months. It was a dark, cold and snowy evening in late October 1974, I was returning to work for just one night a week and I was feeling a little nervous. The arrangement was that my mum and mum-in-law would help Graham out with babysitting in the evenings if need be, and my mum would look after Jonathan during the day following my night shift, while I caught up on sleep and Graham went to work.

I was not eligible to return as a sister, as you had to do a minimum of thirty hours per week for that, so I was back to wearing the pale blue staff midwife uniform I had last worn almost three years earlier. This did not bother me in the slightest. I'd inevitably lost a bit of confidence while being on maternity leave, and my focus was on getting back into the swing of things, not worrying about what rank I was. I would work between the antenatal, labour and postnatal wards, depending where I was needed, and once I had found my feet I planned to increase my hours to two nights per week.

Walking in through the front entrance to the maternity unit at 8.45 p.m., in time for my 9 p.m. start, I felt my nerves start to ease. The distinctive pear-drop smell that always permeated the hospital filled my nostrils, immediately flooding me with a calming feeling of nostalgia and belonging. The clatter of trolleys, the bustle of ambulancemen wheeling patients through the foyer and the distant cries of babies all sounded so familiar I immediately felt at home.

Of course, the last time I had entered the maternity unit was when I was in labour myself, but that all seemed like something of a blur now; practically an event that happened to another version of myself. Then, I don't think I was in any state to notice how the place smelled or looked or sounded. Now I was fully alert again, back on my feet in a new staff midwife uniform that my mum had collected for me from the laundry room the week before, and I was raring to go.

With each step I took across the thick linoleum flooring I could feel my confidence lifting, the worries I felt being replaced by welcome waves of anticipation. The whole maternity unit felt alive and kicking. I could sense it pulsing and bulging with life. Midwives, paramedics and porters were moving in all directions, wearing an assortment of white, green and blue coats and uniforms.

On the way to the night office, where I would be allocated a ward, I spotted Barry, the jovial ambulanceman who had been on the scene a few years earlier when one of my patients went to the toilet and delivered her baby in a plastic washing-up bowl. Memorably, I'd not believed Barry when he told me the baby was coming any minute, and I recalled how my face burnt with embarrassment when it dawned on me that he had been right, and I should have rushed to the patient's aid sooner rather than finishing my cup of tea as I did.

'Evening Nurse!' Barry called to me now, looking at his watch and adding cheekily: 'Off on a tea break are we?'

I didn't mind his teasing at all. I burst out laughing, and it was just the reception I needed. It told me I had history here. People knew me, and I had not been forgotten. Midwife Linda Buckley was back!

I headed to the labour ward, or the 'central delivery suite' as it was now known, on the ground floor. Walking there I saw several heavily pregnant women on trolleys and in wheelchairs. Their cries and moans mingled with the hum of anxious fathers keeping each other company on the corridors. The men were cloistered in shrouds of swirling grey smoke, which mixed with the smell of talc and freshly washed laundry that now filtered through my nostrils.

I heard a newborn baby cry, and it gave me a lump in my throat. A new life had just emerged, and I felt so moved. Just being there, ready for work in my uniform, made me feel excited and important. It was a reminder of what a privilege it is to hear a baby cry for the very first time, assuredly announcing its arrival into the world. I'd missed the adrenaline rush that being on the labour ward gave me, as well as that incredible feeling of being at the start of something new and important and life-changing.

I thought of Jonathan, sleeping soundly in his blue cotton nightie in his cosy cot at home, and I hoped the newborn baby I had just heard cry was as perfect and healthy as my own son.

'Nurse Buckley! It's good to see you again,' Sister Norris said warmly, looming before me with a thick stack of notes in her hand. 'Welcome back. We are *very* glad to have you back. If you thought it was busy before, my oh my, you should see it now!'

'I'm glad to be here,' I replied emphatically.

I felt the very last little knot of nervous tension slip away as I put on a plastic apron and pinned a paper cap on my head. Joyce Norris was the night Sister. She hailed from Jamaica and was an extremely hard worker who expected her staff to be as industrious as she was. If you pulled your weight she liked and admired you, but woe betide you if you didn't. I had never had a problem with her when I'd worked with her occasionally in the past. I preferred to be busy as it meant the shift never dragged, so her reputation as something of a hard taskmaster didn't worry me in the slightest. I was as eager as Sister Norris to crack on with the work.

'You can start with Mrs Grant,' Sister Norris instructed, handing me some notes. 'She's been in the first-stage room for three hours and is just being moved into Delivery Room Five. I've asked a consultant to take a look at her, as her baby appears very large. She may need an assisted delivery.'

'Right away,' I answered, my eyes falling gratefully on the notes. I was flattered to be thrown straight back in at the deep end. It was a vote of confidence from Sister Norris to assign me to what sounded like a potentially difficult delivery on my very first shift back.

I arrived in Room Five to find Dr Bedford washing his hands at the sink. He had clearly just arrived and looked up and greeted me politely, though I'm not sure he instantly recognised me as one of his former patients. I didn't blame him. My pregnancy had been routine, and his presence was not required at the birth, so in the event I had only seen him in the antenatal clinic. I suppose he saw so many women, and I hadn't actually encountered him for over a year now. I was quite relieved, actually, as right at this moment I wanted to be treated as a professional colleague, nothing else.

'It seems Mrs Grant could be expecting rather a large delivery today,' Dr Bedford said. He smiled over at Mrs Grant, who gamely gave a little smile back. It was good to see that Dr Bedford's bedside manner was as warm and comforting as ever. He intimated that I could step in and palpate Mrs Grant's abdomen, saying he would value my opinion. I knew he was preparing to perform a vaginal examination to assess the size of Mrs Grant's pelvis, in view of the size of her baby. Most women didn't object to being examined by a male doctor, but the very idea that an important man like a consultant was required to attend their delivery could alarm a labouring mother unnecessarily.

For that reason, after introducing myself to Mrs Grant and explaining that I was just going to have a feel of her bump, I also went on to tell her exactly what Dr Bedford was going to do, so she understood how his findings might affect the way we managed her delivery.

I could see that she was a naturally slim and petite woman, though her abdomen was absolutely enormous. Mrs Grant winced stoically through her strong contractions as I set about palpating her stomach and examining her. Her skin was pulled as tight as a drum around her bump, making her belly button stick out like the knot of an over-inflated balloon.

I agreed that this baby was indeed on the large side, though Mrs Grant was actually only thirty-seven weeks pregnant and could have gone another three weeks until her due date. I thought it was a jolly good thing she hadn't, or I dreaded to think how big her baby might be, though I kept that to myself.

Mrs Grant's waters had broken when she was taking her toddler to school the day before and she'd been in very slow labour ever since, but it had been stopping and starting at intervals. Dr Bedford proceeded with the examination. He always paid great attention to the patient's dignity, and I admired him for his wonderful manner.

Following the examination he reassured the patient and then had a discreet, hushed conversation with me about the potential use of forceps. I smiled, knowing Mrs Grant was indeed safe in his very capable hands. Dr Bedford went on to reassure *me* he would be on standby to help manage the delivery, given the size of the patient compared with the size of her baby.

It was left to me to explain to Mrs Grant that we might need to put her legs in lithotomy.

'What's that, nurse?' she asked, looking worried.

'It's just stirrups,' I reassured. 'It means we can help support your lower legs, which will give us better access if baby needs a bit of help to come out.'

'Right you are,' she nodded, exhaling deeply.

There was no rush to set up the lithotomy poles, as I anticipated Mrs Grant might still have several hours to go. Dr Bedford had said she was seven centimetres dilated and her labour had been steady, but progress was still fairly slow.

As Mrs Grant applied Vaseline to her lips, which were cracked and dry because of all her deep breathing, I updated her notes and wrote: 'Details of a potential assisted delivery and the need for lithotomy position had been explained to the patient.'

'How are you feeling?' I asked, sitting beside her bed. Dr Bedford had left us to it, promising to call back in as soon as he could, though he had been called to another more urgent delivery.

'Not bad. Not too bad, Nurse.'

Mrs Grant's belly was so big the foetal heart monitor kept slipping off each time she had a contraction, but thankfully I'd managed to keep it in place just long enough to hear that the baby's heartbeat was regular and strong.

'Phhhhhhooooooooooow,' Mrs Grant blew as her abdomen tightened. She was incredibly restrained, and the time began to slip by quickly as she continued to puff and blow in an impressively dignified manner throughout her relentless contractions.

Mrs Grant told me her in-laws ran a confectionary business in Manchester, and that she and her husband hoped to take it over in the future. 'Maybe this little one will keep up the family tradition, too,' she said. 'I hooooooooo … I hope so.'

I chatted easily to Mrs Grant. She seemed very level-headed and was doing a wonderful job working through the pain with just a shot of Pethidine, injected in her buttock. This was the normal place to give it and most women were so well padded in that area they barely felt the needle, but Mrs Grant was so slender I could tell she felt the injection go in. She frowned and gasped a bit, but she didn't complain.

In the shorter and shorter gaps between contractions, Mrs Grant chatted about the fact that she had only recently moved to the area from a tiny village in Derbyshire. 'Don't expect you've heard of it,' she said. 'It's called Parsely Hay and I don't think they have many midwives out there!'

'Can't say I have,' I replied. 'Sounds lovely, though. I do like to go on drives out to the countryside. Perhaps I'll go with my husband one day.'

'Got any children?'

'Yes, just the one, Jonathan. He's ten months old.'

'Ahh, that's nice, Nurse. You don't look like you've just had a baby – I hope I snap back to my size tens like you.'

'I shouldn't think you'll have much trouble,' I replied. 'It looks like you're all bump to me.'

By the time Mrs Grant told me she felt ready to push, three whole hours had passed.

'I have to push right now!' she said. She wasn't in lithotomy yet, and I hoped we wouldn't need it. I pressed the buzzer to summon help, and thankfully Dr Bedford arrived in an instant, just as I was preparing to guide Mrs Grant through her first push.

'OK, on the next contraction … if you could just give me one big push, Mrs Grant …'

'I can. I can … here it is, uuuuurrrgh! Poof pooof poooof.'

'I can see baby's head. You are doing ever so well. Can you give me another one?'

'I can. I caaaargh!'

'Well done! Now wait a bit, wait a bit, until I tell you to push again.'

I decided at this point to perform an episiotomy, because I knew that Mrs Grant would most likely sustain a deep tear if I did not. I infiltrated the perineum with lignocaine so she would not feel the procedure.

I could see Dr Bedford in my peripheral vision, but thankfully I didn't need his help. The baby's head delivered beautifully and I checked that the cord was not around the baby's neck. Everything was going well, so far. Sometimes large babies suffer shoulder dystocia, meaning their shoulders get stuck in the birth canal once the head is already delivered. This can be very dangerous and I was praying I would see first one little pink shoulder, then the next, any moment now.

'Right then, Mrs Grant, go now! Give me a big push now.'

'Uuuurrrggghhhhhhhhhh!'

'Well done, you're doing really well – you've done it!'

Everything happened exactly as it should. The baby gave a little rotation at just the right time, and out she popped, giving a piercing cry as I lifted her up from beneath her armpits and declared: 'It's a girl!'

'Oh, look at her,' Mrs Grant gasped. 'Just look at her.'

I looked at the baby and could only think of one thing: 'She's a whopper!' I thought. I had an idea the baby girl must be well over ten pounds, and Mrs Grant had done a magnificent job delivering such a large baby naturally, without the need for forceps.

'Congratulations,' Dr Bedford said warmly to Mrs Grant. 'Always a pleasure when my services are not required.'

When I weighed the baby, I found that she was actually ten pounds, eight ounces – one of the biggest babies I had ever delivered.

'I would like to congratulate you too, Nurse Buckley,' Dr Bedford said. 'I'm afraid I didn't make the connection straight away, but many congratulations on the birth of your own child, as well as for delivering Mrs Grant's baby so expertly.'

I blushed. I'm not sure if he realised it was my very first day back after maternity leave, and I couldn't quite believe it myself. I thanked him for his kind words and felt absolutely magic. I hadn't experienced a buzz like this since Jonathan had been born.

All that I had to do now was ask one of the other doctors to suture Mrs Grant's perineum following the episiotomy. Nowadays midwives do the stitching themselves after performing an episiotomy, which is much better for the patient and the midwife, but back then a doctor had to do it. I put Mrs Grant in lithotomy to assist the procedure, but unfortunately it took the doctor quite some time to do the suturing, and Mrs Grant's legs were in the lithotomy position for over half an hour. She did not complain, however, as she was too enthralled with her baby girl.

Seeing a delighted Mrs Grant being wheeled off to the post-natal ward some time later, where her bouncing daughter, Christina, was being bathed and dressed in the biggest nightie the staff could find, was a lovely sight. Mrs Grant was positively glowing with happiness, and I absolutely loved being back at work.

I really enjoyed catching up with my colleagues, too. Occasionally I'd be lucky enough to see old friends like Judith Houghton or Barbara Lees, at the shift change-over, although my colleagues generally changed from week to week because of different shift patterns. I'd often find myself on a tea break with a midwife, staff nurse or an auxiliary I didn't know very well. New faces came and went all the time, but we were never short of conversation. Most of the time we'd talk about simple things like knitting patterns, shopping or what we'd done with our husbands and children the week before.

Midwives are very good at chatting, I guess because when you're looking after a labouring mum you have no idea if you'll be together for twenty minutes or twelve hours. Part of the job is to keep communicating in a way that keeps your patient's mind off the pain, but isn't too demanding.

It was the same principle on nights, and I always enjoyed a gentle chitchat with colleagues, particularly if it was a quiet night. Debating anything taxing rarely appealed in the dead of night or the small hours of the morning, especially as we were constantly on standby even during breaks, knowing a new arrival might come in at any moment. That's why knitting patterns were often the hot topic of conversation – however boring that might sound!

In my second week back at work I arrived for my shift to find a tray of twenty-four cakes had been delivered to the labour ward, with my name on it and a thank you note.

'Dear Nurse Buckley, thank you for delivering Christina. Please accept these as a small token of my appreciation, they are from my father's shop. Kind regards, Paula Grant.'

'Oh, that's nice!' I said, passing the tray around and telling Mavis and Betty, two of my favourite auxiliaries, to help themselves if they wanted to take a cake or two home.

As I spoke a young man dressed from head to toe in leather biker's gear came storming into the ward. He tore off his helmet in a panic before blurting out, 'My girlfriend's in labour! Come quick! She's in the corridor! She can't walk any further!'

The doors of the labour ward were swinging open behind him, and through them I could see a heavily pregnant young woman, who was also dressed in black leather trousers and a leather biker's jacket. She began to scream loudly, pushing her back up against the wall and buckling at the knees, looking as if she was about to collapse in agony on the floor. I couldn't see her face as she still had a bright red bike helmet on, emblazoned with a transfer declaring: 'Evel Knievel – Daredevil Legend!' in black-and-gold lettering.

'Let's find you a bed quickly,' I said, putting my arm around her on one side while her boyfriend supported her on the other. 'What's your name?'

'She's called Sally,' the boyfriend said. 'Sally Black.' A blast of hot breath escaped from the helmet as he lifted her visor.

Her face was contorted with pain, and Sally greeted me with a deafening howl.

'Hello, Sally,' I soothed. 'We'll get you comfortable in a moment.'

I wanted to get that helmet off, but it was the least of our worries and that task would have to wait until we'd got her on a bed. We steered Sally tentatively into a first-stage room, which Mavis directed us to, having run ahead as fast as her little legs would carry her. She fetched me a delivery pack as she did so, anticipating I might need it. Mavis was always willing to help, and I knew from the time she assisted me in the birth of a baby in the hospital car park that she particularly enjoyed the drama of a quick, unscheduled delivery.

'Do you need me?' Mavis asked hopefully.

'Yes, please stay,' I said.

From the look of her I suspected Sally was well beyond the first stage, but this was the nearest free room available. Every movement made this poor girl stoop and yelp and wail. The second we got her on the bed she screamed that she wanted to push, and I yanked off her leather trousers as fast as possible. It wasn't too difficult. There were so few maternity clothes on the market in the Seventies and women tended to either swathe themselves in big tents of dresses as I had done, buy clothes a couple of sizes too big, or leave zips and buttons undone.

By the looks of it Sally had squeezed herself into a pair of black leather biker trousers that belonged to her boyfriend. They were only partly zipped up and were wedged underneath her bump and held up with a belt. As soon as I unfastened the belt Sally's abdomen rose like an over-inflated helium balloon.

I instinctively reached for my scissors, to cut her underwear off. It took me right back to the time I delivered baby Keith Miller in the car park, also with trusty Mavis by my side. Just like with Keith, the baby's head was already visible, and as soon as I removed Sally's underwear she grunted and pushed, and there was the baby's head.

'Take your time now, Sally, take some deep breaths, we don't want the baby to come out too quickly.'

'Can't 'elp it, Nurse. Sorry, can't stop … eeeuuurrrgh!'

With that she gave a mighty push and her baby landed neatly on the bed between her legs. The little boy seemed to look me straight in the eye as I dried him off, and then he began to cry heartily. I instinctively looked at Sally's face to see her reaction, and I saw she was smiling and sobbing … inside her motorbike helmet!

'Oh my goodness! The helmet!' I laughed. 'Let's get it off quick!'

'Ralph!' she said through the open visor. 'Help me! I'm boiling me 'ead off!'

He obliged as I proceeded to deliver the placenta and check the baby over. He was a very chubby boy, but fortunately Sally had not torn despite delivering a big baby so rapidly, and without any pain relief whatsoever.

'Are the leathers all right?' she asked Ralph as she gazed lovingly at her new son.

'Yes, right as rain. I'll 'ave 'em back now, but I'll let ya borrow 'em next time.'

Sally groaned playfully and rolled her eyes. 'Next time, my arse,' she said. 'I'll tell ya this for nothin', if there is a next time I'm taking me bleedin' helmet off first. Any chance of a cuppa, Nurse? I got a bit parched in there.'

I found out later, when I visited Sally and baby Carl on the postnatal ward, that she had actually travelled about two miles from Dukinfield to the hospital on the back of her boyfriend's motorbike, her contractions becoming worse at every junction.

'I've never clung onto Ralph so tight before, I tell ya!' she laughed. 'Mind you, I could only just reach round 'im with this little bruiser in the way.' She kissed the top of Carl's soft head.

'Did you not think of calling an ambulance?' I asked.

'Nah, knew it weren't far and we'd be quicker on the bike. Ralph took it dead slow, especially on the corners. We didn't have any change for the phone in any case. 'Appen it was a blessing, else I might have had the baby in the ambulance.'

I couldn't imagine what they must have looked like, navigating the streets of Dukinfield and Ashton with Sally labouring on the back of a motorbike, but it didn't matter now. Carl had arrived safely, and that was the most important thing.

'Can I just check one thing?' I asked as I said goodbye. 'How are you planning to get home?'

Sally looked at me, deadpan, and replied, 'Back o' bike of course, Nurse.' She then erupted with laughter and added cheekily, 'Me dad's coming in his van, don't worry! Me mam's got us a new carrycot and Carl will travel home in style, on the back seat with me.'

'That's good,' I smiled. I knew she wouldn't put the baby on the back of the bike, but if there was anything this job had taught me, it was to always expect to be surprised. I just had to hear for myself that Carl would be transported safely home, and then I could go home happy.

Just as I was about to walk out of the postnatal ward and return to the labour ward, an anxious-looking new mum I'd never met before called me over.

'Nurse, I hope you don't mind, but can I ask your advice?'

'Of course. How can I help?' I asked. She was in the bed nearest the entrance doors, and was holding her tightly swaddled baby close to her chest.

'I don't want to be a nuisance, but I was wondering if I could move to another bed. You see, I can feel a draught through those doors and I'm worried about Lorraine catching a chill.'

I looked at the baby, snug and content inside her soft white blanket, and felt a real connection to her anxious mother, Janet. Little Lorraine was clearly being very well-looked-after and the postnatal ward was not draughty at all. In fact, we always made sure it was always extremely warm and cosy in there.

'Can I have a little hold?' I asked, and Janet carefully passed her precious bundle to me. I held the baby close, too, and rocked her a little in my arms as I spoke to her mum. I couldn't feel a draught, I told Janet. Lorraine was perfectly warm and was not in danger of catching a chill. I could see she was a very much loved little girl, and I told Janet there was really no need to worry.

After I handed the baby back I sat and chatted to Janet for several minutes, reassuring her that she was doing a good job of looking after her baby.

'Thanks, Nurse, it's just good to know that, well, you know, I'm not doing anything wrong, or putting Lorraine in danger or anything like that. Thank you.'

When I finally left the ward I remembered something Sister Kelly had said to me before I had Jonathan.

'I think having a baby yerself can only make yer an even better little midwife,' she had told me.

At the time I didn't take her remark seriously, partly because Sister Kelly did not have children of her own, but now I understood. Being a mother doesn't make you any better at being a professional midwife and delivering babies, but it does help you have a better understanding of what's going on in a new mother's head.

Before, I probably would have swiftly but politely reassured Lorraine's mother that the postnatal ward was maintained at an ideal temperature for newborns and there was no cause for concern. Now, though, I knew exactly how it felt to be in charge of a vulnerable new life. I knew that a mother's fears, however unfounded, should be carefully listened to and not brushed aside. I would hold every new baby that bit tighter now I had my own, because I knew more than ever how incredibly precious each and every baby is, especially to its mum.

Chapter Six

*'Mind if I have a ciggie,
only I'm really nervous?'*

When Jonathan was two and a half years old Graham and I split up, which probably comes as something of a surprise. It certainly came as quite a shock to me at the time. I thought we would always be together, and I couldn't believe what was happening. With the benefit of hindsight, I can see now how we reached the end, although the events I'm about to describe were certainly not clear to me at the time.

Once I'd returned to work and we'd established our weekly routine, Graham and I discovered that going out as a couple was inevitably more complicated with a baby to consider.

'You go to the pub with your friends,' I'd often say. 'I'm fine at home.'

This was perfectly true. Both of our mothers were very willing babysitters should we need them, but I absolutely adored being a mum and was happier at home than anywhere else. Working one day a week gave me a very generous helping of the outside stimulus I needed. I always felt like I'd packed about three days into my one, ten-hour night shift, and the diversity of people I met and experiences I shared were always a marvellous tonic.

I loved my job almost as much as I loved being a mum, and I thought I had my life completely worked out. On my days off I'd shop, see my parents, go to a nursery group or feed the ducks with Jonathan, sometimes with other mums from the neighbourhood.

I enjoyed regular nights out with my old school friends Sue Smith, Susan Thornley and Angela Faulkner, too, a tradition we've kept up to this day. We'd chat about everything from the miners' strike to how the Watergate scandal toppled President Nixon, or what we thought about the new Swedish pop group called ABBA. They'd won the 1974 Eurovision song contest with 'Waterloo', and they wore outlandish, sparkly stage clothes like we'd never seen before.

I'd started to enjoy listening to Tamla Motown music and was keen on Diana Ross and Stevie Wonder at this time. I also liked Barry Manilow and loved singing along to his popular songs like 'Mandy' and 'Could It Be Magic'. Whenever I went out with 'the girls', as we always called ourselves, we'd talk about the latest records we'd bought and compliment each other on the clothes we wore. Jeans were popular then, and I had a pair that fitted so tightly around the hips I had to lie on the floor to zip them up. They had wide flares at the bottom, complete with floral material sewn into the pockets and embroidery around the waistband and hem.

Between us, the girls and I typically paraded a gaudy collection of ponchos, woven handbags, midi-length skirts, platform boots and tie-die tops. Wedged heels and slingback shoes were very popular, too, and we often wore tank tops with floral blouses underneath. We thought we looked the bee's knees, especially when we were dolled up with blue pearlescent eye shadows and bronzing powder on our cheekbones, which replaced our old pots of rouge.

Sometimes we'd have meals in each other's houses. We were all very house-proud and I was thrilled that I had a pampas-coloured bathroom suite that the others were very envious of. Similarly, Angela had an automatic washing machine while the rest of us had twin tubs, so Sue, Susan and I were green with envy about that. Even though we were all interested in what was going on in the world around us, I must admit that we nearly always ended up talking mainly about our husbands and families, or the next holiday or haircut we might have.

Graham and I used to have regular dinner parties with two other couples we were friendly with at that time. We all had young children so we had plenty in common, and we each took it in turn to host the dinners in our homes and prepare adventurous new dishes. Whenever it was my turn to be the hostess I used to make a big effort even though I'm not a fancy cook, and I'd often try out recipes from *The Graham Kerr Cookbook*, which was written by the television chef known as the 'Galloping Gourmet'. I'd received the book as a birthday present, I think.

I remember rustling up dishes like melon and orange for starters, Beef Stroganoff or a cheese fondue for the main course, and Baked Alaska or Rum Baba for dessert. Prawn cocktail starters and Black Forest gâteau were all the rage then, too. The men usually drank beer, and sometimes our guests would bring a Watney's Party Seven keg containing seven pints, which the men would all share, and perhaps a bottle of Blue Nun or Mateus Rosé for the ladies. I have never drunk very much and in those days women generally drank far less than they do today. I might politely sip a little Martini or Cinzano, but I was equally happy drinking fruit punch or a flavoured soda water I mixed up with our Sparklets soda siphon.

There are a few warning signs I can recall leading up to my separation from Graham. We never really argued; it was more a question of us communicating less and less, and then barely at all. In effect, from the time Jonathan was about twelve months old, we seemed to start living quite separate lives, in fact. I remember the timing clearly because in January 1975 I was dismayed to be called to Miss O'Neil's office to discuss a letter of complaint the hospital had received against me, and I did not discuss this with Graham even though it upset me a lot.

'A patient is claiming she was left in lithotomy for too long, and has suffered damage to her back as a result,' Miss O'Neil explained plainly, scanning a letter embossed with the gold crest of a fancy law firm. I'd never had any patient complain about me before, and this took my breath away.

'There is no need to worry,' Miss O'Neil went on. 'I have her file here, and I am very glad to say that your note taking is exemplary, Nurse Buckley. We will have to respond, of course, but I am confident this patient does not have a case.'

'Who is she?' I asked nervously, my throat tight in my neck.

'A Mrs Paula Grant. I'm sure you will recall she had a baby daughter, Christina, weighing ten pounds, eight ounces, last October.'

I could scarcely believe my ears. This was the very same lady who had sent a tray of cakes to the ward to say thank you to me! I remembered every detail of her delivery, of course, as it was the very first one I dealt with upon my return from maternity leave just three months earlier, not to mention the fact Mrs Grant had delivered such a large baby.

'I am shocked,' I stuttered before explaining to Miss O'Neil about the cordial atmosphere in the delivery room, and the thank you gift sent up to the labour ward.

'I clearly remember her being in lithotomy for half an hour. I don't understand.'

'Nurse Buckley, I do not doubt you for one moment. Your notes are very clear and concise. If every midwife practised as you do I'd be extremely happy. I had to notify you of the complaint, but I will deal with the matter. I am confident that once I have circulated copies of your notes to Mrs Grant's solicitor, that will be an end to it.'

It was hectic on the ward for the rest of my shift and I didn't speak to anyone about the matter. Even if I'd had the opportunity, I didn't want to discuss it. To have a complaint directed at me, however unjustified, had given me a very bad taste in my mouth and I felt embarrassed about it even though I knew I was certainly not guilty of any malpractice.

'You all right, love?' Graham asked when I saw him the next day, after he finished work.

I'd slept extremely badly during the daytime and must have looked washed out as I tried to feed a crotchety Jonathan a bowl of stewed apple.

'Fine.' I replied flatly. 'There's some tea in the pot if you want some.'

'No, thanks. I'm meeting the lads for a pint in the Wagon and Horse shortly. Just going to nip up and get changed. Is that turtleneck top of mine ironed?'

Looking back, that was a big moment for me. It signalled the end of the days when I unloaded regularly on Graham, relating every detail of conversations I'd had at work, or babies I'd delivered. I didn't want his opinion any more, but worse than that, I didn't need him, even in a time of trouble.

As I'd matured, my self-confidence had grown and I needed Graham's support less and less. It was natural, I suppose, but this complaint was out of the ordinary, and it had really rattled me. It pained me just to think about it and, despite Miss O'Neil's reassurances, I would not feel exonerated until the case was officially closed. I didn't think Graham could say anything that would make me feel any better and so I kept quiet, and I actually felt relieved when he'd gone out. Our closeness had gone, and I was happier on my own, although we would stay together for another eighteen months.

In the summer of 1975 Graham and I went away for a few days to Norfolk without Jonathan, and I missed him dreadfully. It was mid-August and Jonathan was twenty months old, a stage I was thoroughly enjoying as he was beginning to talk and had just started to walk, after being content to shuffle around on his bottom up until then. I couldn't wait to have his first pair of shoes fitted, and whenever he said 'mum-mum' and put his chubby little hand in mine, my heart completely melted.

'Why ever did I agree to this?' I complained to Graham as we floated down a canal on a barge at an irritatingly slow pace. 'I would never have come away on this stupid trip if you hadn't nagged me into it.'

This was unfair of me. Graham never forced me to do anything against my will; I was just cross with myself for being talked into something I now bitterly regretted. I remember sitting miserably on the barge and listening to 'Sailing' by Rod Stewart on a small transistor radio. The song had just entered the hit parade, as we called it, and I really liked it. On this occasion it made me cry, though, as I thought about my baby at home, being looked after by his grandmother. My mum had recently given up her part-time job in the hospital, having reached retirement age, and would be doing a marvellous job of looking after her grandson. I knew this, but it didn't make me miss Jonathan any less.

The next day the air was very arid and I recall trying to reason with myself as I sat uncomfortably in the blazing sun, shading my head under a big orange-and-purple floppy cotton hat and sipping a glass of fizzy dandelion and burdock. I was wearing a new pair of white high-waist shorts that showed off my tanned legs, and a pretty cheesecloth blouse that tied fashionably in a bow around my middle.

I told myself to think how fortunate I was compared with others. The Vietnam War had ended a few months earlier, in April 1975, and I thought of the dreadful suffering that had been inflicted on so many innocent people. As I'd packed the suitcases for our holiday, I'd heard on the television news that six men had been jailed for life (wrongly, as we now know) for the Birmingham pub bombings that killed twenty-one people in November 1974, the month after I'd returned to work. My upset at being separated from Jonathan for a few days was absolutely nothing when I thought about the misery IRA atrocities and the Troubles in Northern Ireland brought to others.

'Come on, Linda,' I told myself as I rubbed some coconut oil into my skin. 'Jonathan is fine. Try to relax, you'll be home tomorrow.'

Still, that night I pushed Graham away, angry I couldn't cuddle my son and kiss him goodnight. I was very relieved when we finally pulled up the drive at home and I turned the key in our front door again. Holding Jonathan, all warm and snug and smelling of mashed banana and baby soap, made me want to cry with happiness.

I was aware that Graham and I were spending less time together as he went out more and more in the evenings, but it didn't bother me, and at the time I didn't see the danger in that. My focus was on bringing up Jonathan and doing my best at work. If I'm honest, my job enriched my life a great deal more than my marriage did at that time. Without consulting Graham I had my hair cut short at a little salon in Stockport, as I thought it would be easier to manage, even though he had always loved my long hair.

Now it's so obvious to look back and see we were on a slippery slope, but it would take another year for us to actually split up, in the steamy, heat-wave summer of 1976. When the end came, I'd had a particularly hectic few weeks at work, delivering at least five babies during each long night shift throughout June. On one particularly humid evening I snatched a break in the day room at around 10 p.m., where the talk was all about the plague of ladybirds and the water shortage the unusually hot weather had brought.

'Have yer seen those stickers in all the cars?' Sister Kelly had remarked earlier to me and Stella, who was now fully qualified. '"Save Water, Bath With a Friend" they say. I ask yer!'

Stella and I both chuckled and shared a knowing glance. It would have been too unkind to say it, but I didn't expect the water shortage would have affected Sister Kelly too much in any case, as she certainly didn't have a reputation for being the most hygienic member of staff.

The hospital itself was not subject to water restrictions, but I remember the grounds of the maternity unit looking scorched and brown instead of green, and the collection of Datsun Sunnys, Ford Capris and Morris Marinas in the car park were thick with dust because hosepipe and car-washing bans were in place across the country. Even some of the Tarmac pavements had melted, it was that hot.

I drank down a large tumbler of orange squash and was fanning myself with a 'Save Water!' leaflet when Sister Norris put her head round the door.

'There you are, Nurse Buckley,' she said. 'Take this one, please. Janice Povey. She's in the admissions room.'

Sister Norris handed me a bundle of notes and I got to my feet immediately and went to find the patient. Janice was twenty-eight years old and, at first glance, appeared to be labouring very well. When I asked if she had anyone with her she shook her head emphatically, and I noticed she was not wearing a wedding ring.

'I was at work when me waters went in the toilet,' she explained, gesturing towards the blue tabard apron that covered her clothing.

'I work in a bingo hall, as a cleaner. I just got in a taxi, on me own, like, and came straight here.'

'That's fine,' I replied. 'There's a pay phone you can use before we get you in the labour room, if you'd like to let someone know you're here. Let's have a look how far along you are.'

Janice nodded uncertainly before wincing and clutching her abdomen as it tightened. 'Ooooh, that were right nasty. Mind if I have a ciggie, only I'm really nervous?'

'No, I'm sorry you can't, it's really not encouraged on the wards.'

Janice's apron and the saggy polyester dress she wore beneath it smelled of a mixture of cigarette smoke, stale beer and lavatory cleaner.

'Right,' she huffed and puffed as I set about examining her. 'How long do you think I'll be? It's baking hot in 'ere.'

With that Janice whistled in a long, deep breath as she experienced another strong contraction. She was already six centimetres dilated, I found, and I told her we'd get her into a delivery room very shortly, although of course she might have several hours yet to go. 'Flaming 'eck,' she complained, which became her mantra for the next few hours or so, on and off.

Janice's baby girl was eventually born at just before 4 a.m. the next morning after a perfectly routine labour. Janice did really well, dragging on gas and air and refusing the offer of Pethidine, saying she was 'doin' all right' without it. At one point she even said she was feeling 'champion' in between her grumbles of 'flamin' 'eck', which was not an expression I'd heard a labouring woman use before. I thought there was something not quite right with Janice, actually, as this wasn't the only unusual thing she'd done.

She had not wanted to phone anybody at all, and as far as I was aware nobody knew she had come here straight from work, which was odd. I suspected the problem was that she was not only unmarried, but perhaps she was no longer with the father of her baby. I wasn't sure, though, as she was giving nothing away.

It was still a little unusual in 1976 for a pregnant woman not to be married, or at least 'promised' to someone. If a single women found herself 'in the club', as it was often referred to then, it was not uncommon for a 'shotgun wedding' to be hastily arranged, typically in the register office with the blushing bride wearing a two-piece suit or a fitted off-white dress instead of a flowing white gown.

Sometimes women turned up at the hospital wearing wedding rings when you could see from the notes they were actually a 'Miss'. They clearly didn't want to admit they were having a child out of wedlock and so I would just refer to the partner as her husband to make her feel better. It didn't matter to me what her marital status was; my job was simply to make the woman feel as comfortable as possible in order to deliver her baby safely.

However, being a pregnant woman without a partner at all, as I suspected was Janice's predicament, was really quite rare for a twenty-eight-year-old at that time. It was typically only the trickle of pregnant young teenagers we saw who were not only single, but completely on their own. Nevertheless, I treated Janice exactly as I would any other patient, and tried to make her feel at ease by chatting to her and showing an interest in her life.

Janice remained cagey, though, and even avoided telling me which bingo hall she worked in. 'Oh, you wouldn't know it,' she said, closing her eyes, as she had done every time she wanted to steer the conversation in another direction.

Her healthy little girl weighed eight pounds exactly, had an extremely good pair of lungs on her and was splattered in blood and sticky vernix when she made her entrance into the world. She cried loudly as I attempted to clean her up using cotton wool swabs, and she didn't stop until she was neatly swaddled in an NHS blanket and lying comfortably on her side in a cot.

We'd recently had the luxury of receiving some samples of disposable nappies at the hospital, which we midwives thought were a marvellous improvement on the old terry towelling ones. Disposable wipes and protective bed sheets were also welcome new supplies at this time, and they made us whoop with glee the first time we saw them. However, we were under strict instructions not to give the nappies or wipes out 'willy-nilly' but to use them sparingly, to test out what we thought of them and to gauge what the women themselves thought. I think the nappy companies were using midwives for free market research, which was fine by us.

'I've put a terry nappy on your daughter, but I can let you have a few disposable nappies if you like,' I said. I wanted to engage Janice in conversation, and I also imagined she would be very grateful for the offer of a few nappies.

'Whatever', she replied impassively and, unlike practically every other new mum I had encountered, did not ask for a cuddle as her daughter lay in the cot at the side of her bed.

After examining the placenta to make sure it was fully intact, as it should be, I finished writing up my notes and tidied up. Janice's placenta was perfectly healthy looking and so I took it down the corridor to a large freezer we had in a side room and deposited it, unwrapped, alongside scores of other placentae. They looked like a lot of big pieces of steak. Some were already deep-frozen, others were partly frozen, having been placed in the freezer more recently. It was routine for midwives to place healthy placentae in this freezer, and we all understood that they were collected by cosmetic companies, who used them to make women's face creams and the like. The oestrogen and progesterone in the placenta were believed to be a valuable and effective addition to beauty products. That's what we understood, and I don't recall any of us midwives ever questioning the practice. It was simply one of those standard routines we were taught from the start and accepted as the norm, and the only placentae that didn't go in the freezer were ones that were incomplete and would need further examination, or were soiled from meconium, which happens when a baby opens its bowels in the womb.

By now a half hour or more had passed since Janice's baby was born. The new mum had said next to nothing, lying quietly with her eyes shut for most of the time.

'Have you thought of any names?' I asked, trying to get her to talk when I noticed her eyes flicker open.

'No,' Janice replied sleepily, shuttering her eyelids back down.

'Oh, well, you can perhaps have a little think when we get you settled on the postnatal ward. I'll be back very shortly; you have a little rest while I get someone to come and move you.'

When I returned just a few minutes later I was dismayed to see that Janice was off the bed and struggling out of her NHS gown. She was attempting to put her own clothes back on, which she'd kept in a carrier bag beside the bed. I told Janice there was really no need to change before we got her on the ward, as most women stayed in their nightdresses and dressing gowns until they were ready to go home, usually two days later.

'I didn't bring an overnight bag,' Janice said flatly. 'What with me coming straight from work, an' all. I've not got a dressing gown, so I'm happier in me own clothes.'

I didn't argue, as the NHS nightgown she was wearing gaped down the back and did not look a comfortable fit, and in fact I helped button Janice into her old floral dress before settling her back on the bed.

'Now I have to just check on another patient,' I told her. 'One of my colleagues will help move you and settle you up on the postnatal ward very soon, and I'll come and see you before I finish my shift.'

Janice nodded appreciatively and even gave me a smile. 'Thanks, Nurse,' she said. 'You've been very kind.'

I dearly wished that when I went up to the ward later Janice would be in a better frame of mind, and hopefully cuddling her baby. However, when I got there at just after 7 a.m. she was nowhere to be seen. I'd been looking after my other patient for an hour or so and knew nothing of the drama that had unfolded in my absence.

'Social Services have been called,' Rita, a new pupil midwife, told me apologetically. 'Miss Povey insisted on leaving, and left the baby behind. There was nothing we could do to stop her …'

I was open-mouthed with amazement. I knew there was something not quite right about Janice, but I didn't imagine for one moment she would do such a thing.

'She put an apron on over her dress,' Rita continued, looking like she might cry. 'She said she had to go, but she'd be back later. She wouldn't listen to me when I said she had to stay. Sister took it from there.'

'Thanks for telling me,' I replied. 'And please don't worry – this is not your fault, you know. If a patient takes it upon herself to walk out of the hospital, unfortunately there's not a lot we can do to stop her.' I rubbed Rita's arm.

I found out later that Janice never did return to the ward as she promised, which didn't surprise anybody. She did subsequently visit her GP, though, who referred her to a community midwife for postnatal care. I eventually learned that Janice never saw her baby again, and asked Social Services to arrange to have the little girl adopted. It seems poor Janice had hidden her pregnancy from everybody, including her employer, and had planned to leave the baby in the hospital all along.

I never got to hear any more than that, and could only guess at what had happened with the father of the child to have forced Janice into such an unfortunate position. I assumed that the father was not a steady partner and probably didn't even know about the baby, but I didn't know for sure. I felt very sorry for Janice and wished she had felt able to open up to me when she was having the baby, as I would have liked to have been able to offer some help, or at least a friendly ear.

The day after this unsettling incident I was sitting on the settee at home, mulling over all this information and wondering if I could have done more to help Janice, when Graham appeared.

I hadn't been expecting him home from work so early, as it was only just after 4 p.m. I could tell immediately something was wrong as he had beads of sweat on his forehead and looked quite agitated. Jonathan was sound asleep in his pram, which I'd placed by the back door in the shade, and I instinctively felt glad he was not in the room with us, as this was not going to be good news.

I can't remember Graham's exact words because I think my brain fogged over. It felt very surreal, but I heard him say the words 'leaving you' and 'it's over.'

'OK, then,' I replied, very coolly. 'If that's what you want. I won't stop you.'

Graham packed up some of his belongings and left within twenty minutes. We didn't fight or even argue, and I didn't break down in tears. Looking back, the scenario seems quite unbelievable, but it was truly that brief and simple. I was shocked, of course, even though I knew the writing had been on the wall as we had drifted apart further and further in recent months. I certainly wasn't heartbroken, though, at least not for myself. Jonathan was my only concern. How would his life be affected by our marriage ending? I knew without having to ask that Graham would still be a part of Jonathan's life. He was a good father, but we were simply no longer a good couple.

I didn't argue with Graham, or even question him, because I knew deep down that there was nothing to fight over. Our relationship had run its course. We'd grown up together since he was sixteen and I was seventeen, but more than a decade had passed since then. Now we were twenty-seven and twenty-eight years old, and both quite different people to the teenagers we once were. In short, we were no longer in love and, perhaps worse than that, I think we felt quite indifferent to each other.

When Graham had gone I cuddled Jonathan and felt a deep pang of sorrow on my little boy's behalf. I told him his father would always love him and he was not leaving *him*, only me. Jonathan was very quiet, and when I stopped talking I was very aware of the silence surrounding us. Graham's voice was not going to cut through the silence as it once might have done. He had gone to stay at his mother's house for the time being. I think that was the saddest moment in the breakdown of my marriage. I didn't like such silence, but I knew I didn't want Graham back. Our marriage had died, and that silence marked its passing.

I remember phoning my own mum quite calmly, and explaining what had happened. My voice cracked a little as I spoke and I felt sorry and a little guilty to be the bearer of bad news, but I also felt an element of relief as I spoke. The news knocked everyone for six, of course. We were perceived as a 'lovely young couple' within the family, and particularly by the friends of my parents who didn't know us that well but had attended our wedding almost seven years earlier.

I reassured my mum that I would be fine, and it was for the best, because I really believed that was true. In typical style, she and my dad both said they would support me and do whatever they could to help me. There was no big drama, and they didn't try to change my mind or interfere.

As the first night alone stretched into a week and then a month and more, I didn't feel lonely. Sadly, I acknowledged that I was no less on my own that when my marriage had been failing, because Graham and I had ended up living such separate lives.

'How will you manage?' I remember a rather nosy neighbour saying to me at a toddler group some weeks later. She looked absolutely horrified as she spoke. 'I'd not cope at all if I were on my own.'

'I'll manage fine,' I replied. 'I *am* managing fine, honestly I am.'

The neighbour was about the same age as me but she reminded me of a younger version of myself: the teenage Linda who needed Graham's support to get through the day. I looked at her and realised just how much I had grown up. I was an independent woman with a good job, and I was perfectly capable of raising my son as a single mother. The prospect didn't worry me at all, and I told her as much. She practically winced when I used the word 'single mother'.

'There are far worse things that can happen,' I said, thinking of some of the very sad situations I had encountered through my work. 'And in my experience things have a habit of working themselves out.'

Chapter Seven

'What an impatient little boy you are!'

I threw myself into my work, and looking after Jonathan, of course. Work was my therapy and it always has been, helping me through other tough times that lay ahead. My mum was fantastic, offering to look after Jonathan more so I could work two nights a week. I would need the extra money after the divorce, which would take about six months to process.

Over the following months, as Graham and I gradually dismantled the life we had built together, dividing old photographs, wedding gifts, furniture and finances, I always looked forward to losing myself in my work. Being in the maternity unit brought me so much joy. It was a pleasure to bring new life into the world instead of dealing with the demise of my marriage.

It was around this time that I had a rather amusing experience whilst delivering a baby. Women who were ten days or more overdue, or whose waters had broken but had not started labouring, were always brought in and induced in the afternoon. They would be given a Prostin pessary containing a hormone to stimulate the cervix and bring the onset of labour. The hope was that it would start to work straightaway, but if it didn't the process would be repeated after six hours and another pessary would be inserted in the vagina. Alternatively, they might have their waters broken and be commenced on a Syntocinon infusion, which also stimulated the onset of labour.

More often than not women who had come in for an afternoon induction delivered their baby during the evening or in the small hours of the morning, which contributed to the high number of deliveries we had during the night shift. Nowadays we do it the other way around, inducing women in the evening in the hope they will deliver during the day, when there are more midwives and doctors available.

It was bonfire night in November 1976 when Sister Norris sent me upstairs to Ward 27, the antenatal ward, with the familiar instruction: 'Nurse Buckley, there's another induction needs bringing down.'

I took the lift to the first floor and found a friendly-faced lady called Lillian Leyton preparing to be moved onto a trolley, upon which she would be wheeled downstairs to the labour ward. Mavis, the auxiliary, was talking to Mrs Leyton ten to the dozen, as she had a habit of doing when she found herself in the thick of the action.

'Hello, Linda!' Mavis waved as I approached the bed. 'Am I glad to see you! This is a fourth baby, you know!'

All midwives, not to mention experienced auxiliaries like Mavis, knew that fourth babies had a tendency to deliver quickly. The same is often true of second babies, although the third child can be trickier and is commonly perceived by midwives as being a more difficult delivery. I've no idea why this is the case, although some midwives have a theory that a woman who has already given birth to two babies expects the third to be easier still. Perhaps this optimistic expectation makes the reality seem worse than it really is? It's the closest I can come to any kind of explanation.

Anyhow, Mrs Leyton was having very regular contractions that were only a couple of minutes apart, and she gave me a welcoming smile. 'Hope this is quicker than last ti – aaar-rrggghh! Than last time.'

It wasn't until that moment that I realised I'd delivered Mrs Leyton's previous baby, a boy called Christopher, when I was pregnant with Jonathan. She'd had a tough time and her very long labour was so painful she had two shots of Pethidine four hours apart before Christopher arrived after a mammoth twelve-hour labour. We'd actually been on the verge of need-ing to administer a third dose of Pethidine, which was very unusual and would have had to be signed off by a consultant. In the end Mrs Leyton had been so exhausted she could barely speak, I recalled.

'Is your husband here this time?' I asked, remembering fondly that he gave her a Fry's Chocolate Cream bar for a much-needed sugar boost last time as she lay flat out on the delivery bed, energy depleted and eyelids drooping.

'I h-h-hope so,' she huffed. 'On 'is w-a-ayyyy.'

'That's good, but let's hope you don't need the chocolate this time! I think things are moving much faster, thank goodness.'

She gave me a sweet smile, but I could see she was now concentrating too much on dealing with her labour pains to join in any further conversation. I always enjoyed encounter-ing former patients again, especially if I was lucky enough to be the one to deliver the sibling of a baby I'd previously helped into the world.

This first started to happen around the time I was pregnant with Jonathan, because the women I delivered as a new pupil midwife in 1970 were ready to have another child two or three years on. They always looked pleased to see a familiar face and

I always tried to mention something positive that happened the last time, to put each woman at ease and to make her feel special, as each and every pregnant lady should.

Sometimes I chatted to the ladies about how the hospital had changed over the years, and Mavis in particular always enjoyed reminiscing. I think she thought it was a comfort to patients to know how familiar she was with the hospital, and how long she had worked there, which was about twenty years.

It was always interesting listening to Mavis. She was very proud of the fact the original Ashton District Infirmary had been in existence since 1861, no less, and once had a separate workhouse built nearby. When the NHS was formed in 1948, the hospital was joined on to the old workhouse building to form the new Ashton-under-Lyne General Hospital. Earlier this year, in 1976, the hospital had been renamed Tameside General Hospital, which came about because of the establishment of Tameside Metropolitan Borough Council a couple of years previously.

'So you've had three babies in Ashton General and the next will be born at Tameside Hospital's maternity unit,' Mavis summed up, grinning at Mrs Leyton. 'You'll have to explain to your children that it's one and the same place!'

I think that was the very last thing on Mrs Leyton's mind, as the contractions were now coming thick and fast. Mavis tried to help me to transfer Mrs Leyton onto a trolley but it took quite a long time and the poor patient stopped and grimaced and clenched her fists tightly with each new ripple of pain.

When she was finally lying down on the trolley we wheeled her into the lift, and a couple of minutes later the three of us – myself, Mrs Leyton, plus a wide-eyed Mavis – were on our way down at last. Mrs Leyton held onto Mavis's arm for dear life as I reached across and pressed the button to close the lift door.

As we descended and approached the ground floor the patient let out an almighty cry that reverberated all around the metal walls. 'It's all right, love,' I heard Mavis soothe as I instinctively lifted the hem of Mrs Leyton's nightdress, to check what was happening down below. To my surprise the baby's head was already starting to bulge through her underwear.

'Now then, let's slip your pants off as I can see the baby is already trying to come.'

'Got – to – PUSH!' Mrs Leyton bellowed as I pulled off her underwear.

'Take your time,' I said. 'Just take your time. Keep breathing. Can you hang on just a minute?'

'OOOOOOhhhhhhhhh, OOOOOOOOOhhhhhh!' she blew, 'Noooo. No. Nooooo!'

I saw her grit her teeth and she fired her baby out with two small, sharp pushes. The slippery baby boy landed on the trolley between Mrs Leyton's legs.

'Aaaaaaarghhhhhhh!' she huffed. 'Have I done it? Have I?' The little boy belted out a loud wail.

'You certainly have!' I replied.

At that precise moment the lift ground to a halt and the metal doors slid open automatically. Mrs Leyton, Mavis and myself all looked up to see a junior doctor in a white coat standing on the corridor, waiting for the lift. He looked back at us in absolute astonishment as the baby continued to a cry from beneath Mrs Leyton's nightgown, which was stretched between her elevated knees and formed a neat little canopy over the noisy little boy.

'Excuse me, please can you let us through?' I said urgently to the young doctor, who very swiftly stepped aside to let us pass.

I covered the baby in a towel Mrs Leyton had in her overnight bag and left him wrapped warmly on the bed, knowing we were just moments away from the delivery room, and deciding it was safer not to lift him up while we were in transit. Then we steered Mrs Leyton very carefully to the nearest free delivery room, where I told her we would deliver the placenta.

'Well done!' Mavis squealed excitedly, rubbing the back of Mrs Leyton's hand as she kept apace with the trolley. 'What a tale you'll have to tell your little lad!'

'I'll say,' I soothed as we settled into a delivery room and I cut the baby's cord, delivered the placenta and weighed him.

Mrs Leyton began to laugh quite uncontrollably when I finally let her hold her son, once he was dressed in a nappy and nightie and wrapped in a clean blanket.

'I don't know! What a drama! What an impatient little boy you are,' she chuckled. 'But look at you, you're gorgeous!'

My heart was full of happiness. This was what life was all about. I loved the unpredictable nature of birth, and I absolutely adored hearing delighted new mothers cooing over their babies. Nothing else mattered to them at that moment in time. Mrs Leyton could have given birth on the street outside and she would have still reacted in this wonderful way, only having eyes for her new baby, and thinking how lucky she was that he had arrived safely.

When I visited Mrs Leyton the next day, she was full of smiles once more, and thanked me over and over again.

'I'm so glad it was you, Nurse,' she said. 'I knew everything would be all right, as soon as I saw you. Here, my husband brought you some treacle toffee. He can't believe our son was born in a lift and he was sorry he missed it, but all's well that ends well, eh?'

'Thanks. And that's a lovely compliment, thank you,' I said.

Mrs Leyton didn't dwell on the fact her baby had been born in the lift, and actually seemed more taken with the fact he was born on Bonfire Night.

'Remember, remember the Fifth of November – how will I ever forget?' she cooed, gently stroking her little boy, Kevin, under the chin.

'My mum said we should have called him Guy, but I prefer Kevin.'

It's often the case that the most extraordinary happenings surrounding a birth become disregarded as soon as the baby arrives. Having a healthy child eclipses everything, even an unconventional birth like this one. No doubt once Mrs Leyton had fully recovered and settled back home, she would regale her friends with the funny story about where she gave birth, and how the junior doctor had the surprise of his life when he called for the lift that night. For now, though, she had much more momentous news in her hands; she had become a mum for the fourth time, and that's what mattered most.

'Why don't you go out with that nice neighbour of yours?' Mum asked one Saturday afternoon. She was peering out of my kitchen window, which looked out onto my garden, and beyond that into the back garden belonging to my neighbour, Ian Fairley. He was a fair-haired policeman and he, too, was recently separated and had a little boy.

'Funny you should say that,' I replied. 'We're taking the boys to the park later.'

Mum beamed. 'That's good, Linda! I don't like to think of you being on your own, and he seems like a very respectable man. He's a good match for you.'

I wanted to roll my eyes but I resisted. Mum didn't know Ian at all, but the fact he was a policeman and he appeared to play a very hands-on role in his young son's life despite being separated from his wife clearly impressed her. I'd agreed to bring Jonathan along and go to Stamford Park at four o'clock with Ian and his son Stuart, who was five years old.

It was November 1976, and I'd been slowly getting to know Ian on and off for a few months. Sometimes he called round for a cup of tea after we'd bumped into each other in the street or at the local shops.

'Come round, it'll be nice for the boys to play together,' I'd say. That was always my safety net. I wasn't looking for a new relationship, and I really wasn't sure about Ian. As a policeman he saw things as very black and white, whereas for a midwife there is always a grey area because we are not dealing with law enforcement, but the very individual art of caring for a woman and delivering her baby.

Today was our first proper outing together and I had to admit I felt slightly nervous, as if I might be on the cusp of starting something new. Though I wasn't looking to settle down again so soon after splitting up from Graham, I did like the idea of having a man in my life once more; someone to talk to and laugh with, but perhaps not much more than that.

Seeing women like Mrs Leyton having her fourth child inevitably made me wonder whether I might have any more children myself one day. I certainly wasn't desperate for this to happen, although I thought it might be good one day, if things worked out for me and I met the right person at the right time. Equally, I felt that if I remained on my own, that would be fine, too. I had a comfortable, uncomplicated life and Jonathan was a happy little boy. After one or two hiccups, Graham and I had fallen into a civilised routine. He saw Jonathan regularly, and I was quite content with the way things had panned out.

When I went to the park with Ian that day, he immediately got me talking about my job, which always puts me at my ease.

'It must be so interesting being a midwife,' he said. 'I suppose it's a bit like being a policeman – you never know what's going to happen from one day to the next. Am I right?'

I knew that Ian was a very principled man and I didn't want to talk about specific deliveries, as this felt too personal. I also thought that perhaps it might have been perceived as being a little unprofessional of me, talking about my patients to someone I didn't know very well at all. However, he was keen to hear more about my job and I decided to tell him about a very memorable birth that had taken place a month or so earlier, which one of my midwife colleagues, Jean, had relayed to me.

I thought Ian would be interested in this story, and that it would give him a good insight into the work of a midwife. We sat on a bench in the park, watching Jonathan and Stuart scamper around the play area as I told the tale.

A twenty-five-year-old woman called Philomena Warren arrived at the unit in the early stages of labour one morning. She was very well spoken and explained that her husband had brought her in but was going to call in at his office to 'tie up a few loose ends' before returning to the hospital.

'He'd like to witness the birth, but I'd prefer it if he didn't,' she confided. 'I don't think it's decent for a man to see his wife in such a way.'

My friend Jean assured Philomena that having the husband present at the birth was actually a very bonding experience for the vast majority of couples, and that more and more men were joining their wives in the delivery room.

'No, it's not for me, thank you,' Philomena said firmly. 'I'd be very grateful if you could keep him out.'

It was almost an hour later when Mr Warren turned up, and Philomena had become very anxious, even though her contractions were still only mild and infrequent. 'Don't let him in!' she ordered Jean when she heard her husband was on the corridor outside. 'I don't want to see him. I don't want him to see me. Please, do whatever you can.'

Philomena's face was as white as a sheet and she had begun biting her neatly manicured nails and chewing on her bottom lip nervously.

'Perhaps he might be a help,' Jean suggested. 'Sometimes husbands are very good at helping their wives stay calm during labour.'

'Out of the question!' Philomena blurted. 'I'm doing this ON MY OWN!'

Several hours passed, during which time Mr Warren sat very dutifully in the corridor waiting for news. This was their first child and they had been married for three years. Jean popped outside to chat with him once or twice, to let him know that his wife was progressing well, if slowly. He didn't question the fact he wasn't allowed into the delivery room, and told Jean that he respected Philomena's wishes.

It turned out Mr Warren was a corporate solicitor. Jean told me this because she laughed about the fact that at one point in the long night she had unexpectedly ended up having a conversation with him at about the Equal Pay Act. Midwives had welcomed the Act with open arms, as of course most women did. However, our profession was so female-dominated we were worried that we might not benefit from it. 'There are no male midwives, not that we know of!' Jean had lamented to Mr Warren. 'So how can we benefit from the Act? How can our pay be matched to that of our male colleagues when we don't have any?'

Jean couldn't remember what Mr Warren's answer had been, and explained that she had only really tried to engage him in conversation to find out a bit more about him. She was concerned about why his presence seemed to make his wife fearful. In Jean's opinion Mr Warren was a thoroughly decent, charming and well-educated man, which only added to the mystery. It wasn't until a full six hours later that the truth emerged, quite literally.

'Linda, I kid you not, I have never been so surprised in my life,' Jean told me. 'Never in a million years would I have predicted what was about to happen.'

Philomena pushed out a baby boy, and to Jean's surprise and Philomena's horror, he was unmistakably of mixed race. The creases in his skin were jet black, and his palms and the soles of his feet were markedly lighter than the rest of his skin.

'Oooh, look, you've got a lovely little boy,' Jean said instinctively despite her shock, because the baby was indeed a very handsome little boy with the most beautiful big, round eyes and long, silky eyelashes. Jean remembers her mouth dropping open, and told me she was sorry she was not wearing a mask over her mouth and nose, as we had done until recently. They'd been phased out as it was decided they did not really do a great deal to stop the spread of infection, and unfortunately for Jean this meant she had nothing to hide her surprised expression behind.

'It's a black baby! That's not mine!' Philomena cried.

'Well it's not mine,' Jean replied, not knowing what else to say. At this point Philomena, who'd inhaled a great deal of gas and air, let out a hoot of incredulous laughter and then burst into tears.

'What will I tell him?' Philomena sobbed. 'I didn't mean for this to happen, for things to go this far … I love my *husband*! What will I do?'

'I think he seems like a very reasonable man,' Jean said. 'Why don't we let him come in, and then we'll see.'

Philomena eventually agreed, after spending about fifteen minutes fretting and trying to compose herself. She had the baby in her arms now, his cute little face peeping out of a pale blue blanket. There was no mistaking he was not a white baby, but Philomena made no excuses when Mr Warren was invited into the room.

'Look,' she said, tilting the little bundle towards her husband, so he could clearly see the baby's face. 'It's a boy.'

Mr Warren behaved like a true gentleman, as Jean had hoped he would. He took a sharp intake of breath and stood silently for a moment, looking intently at the snuffling little boy, but he made no reference whatsoever to the colour of the baby's skin.

'This is my son,' Philomena said, rocking the baby in her arms in the blanket.

Mr Warren stared at his wife and then back at the baby. You could hear them both breathing, it was that quiet in the room.

'I'm glad he's arrived safely,' he said. 'Er, I need some time to think, if you'll excuse me.'

Mr Warren stood up to leave, took two paces towards the door and turned around. He then took the two paces back, leant in and stroked the little boy's cheek tenderly before turning on his heel and walking slowly out of the room.

Ian listened intently to my story. Being a man, I think he was angry on Mr Warren's behalf. 'What happened?' he asked crossly. 'Surely they couldn't carry on as if nothing had happened?'

I didn't know the answer to his question. Jean had heard that Mr Warren certainly stood by his wife in the early weeks, when the community midwife was doing home visits, but what happened in the weeks and months that followed, nobody was sure.

'You see, it's really not like your job at all,' I said to Ian. 'Having babies can be a messy, complicated business, and when things don't go to plan, there is no law about how to deal with it. I think it's best not to apportion blame or try to punish a person for mistakes they've made. The important thing is to do what is best for the baby.'

Ian listened and nodded, but I wasn't sure he really got where I was coming from. I didn't realise it at the time, but I actually said something very profound that day. This distinction between our jobs and the very different worlds we inhabited at work was intrinsically linked to our characters, and that would have a huge bearing on the next fifteen years of my life.

As Ian and I spent more and more time together with Jonathan and Stuart we became very close, despite our differences. Above all else, at that time I think Ian was like a comfort blanket to me. It was actually quite unusual to be a single mother in those days, although I don't remember feeling I had any stigma attached to me and nobody who really knew me judged me.

My work colleagues gave me nothing but support, always asking after Jonathan and making sure I was all right. I appreciated their concern but I didn't want sympathy, or for my private life to be the talk of the wards. I only told the other midwives what I wanted them to hear, which was that we were managing fine, and that I didn't want my husband back so there was no need to worry about me. This was perfectly true, a fact that surprised me and I think rather upset Graham, even though he was the one who had left me. I was happy enough without him, particularly now Ian was on the scene and I was enjoying his company, and not spending so much time on my own.

In those days people didn't really just live together, particularly with children involved, and as Ian liked to do things correctly I wasn't surprised when he proposed just a few months after we got together. There was no romantic gesture; it was more a case of him saying to me one night over a cup of tea, 'I think we should get married and live together. Do you?'

I heard myself saying 'yes' although I couldn't quite believe how quickly things were moving forward. My heart told me to go ahead. I would be able to start a new chapter in my life. Jonathan would be part of a proper little family unit once more and my parents would be very pleased I had settled down again. It was perfect. My head told me this was all happening a little too fast, but ultimately my heart won the day. What was there to be worried about? I had the chance to be happily married again, and I was going to take it, even though I had only been on my own for a few months. The decision was made there and then.

Ian and I married on 29 January 1977 at the register office in Dukinfield, just south of Ashton, and my old school friend Sue was my bridesmaid for the second time. Afterwards about sixteen members of our family and a few close friends had a meal at the Trough Hotel in nearby Droylsden. I wore a velvet crimson jacket and a patterned skirt to match, and Ian wore a navy blue suit. It was a lovely day, and I felt optimistic about the future.

By now I wanted another baby very much. Ian and I had talked about this as we prepared for the wedding, and we were both in agreement that we did not want to wait too long before trying to have a baby together. Jonathan was three by this time, and Stuart nearly six. We made a happy little family, and I have some wonderful memories of our early years together.

I remember the occasion of the Queen's Silver Jubilee, in June 1977, very fondly. The main street in Mottram was sealed off for a street party and there were trestle tables laid out down the middle, and bunting everywhere. I bought souvenir mugs for the boys, and in hospital we had an afternoon tea party for the staff and patients. There was a real 'feel good' factor in the air, which perfectly complemented how I was feeling in my own life. I was coming up to 30, and I was in a good place once more.

By September 1977 I was expecting my second child, and I could not have felt happier.

'I'm proud of how you got your life back on track so quickly,' Mum said when I broke the happy news. 'That's my Linda! Good for you!'

Everyone was happy, it seemed. I'd sold my house and moved into Ian's smart, detached home, and by now Stuart was living with us full time. Stuart and Jonathan shared a bedroom and got along well together. We enjoyed family day trips and I used to love driving to Abersoch in North Wales in a little Mini Clubman we owned. We did that trip when I was heavily pregnant, so it must have been around Easter 1978, with the baby due in June.

'Wouldn't it be lovely if we had a little girl?' I said to Ian as we watched the boys run along the sand, licking the Zoom ice lollies we bought for ninepence each at the café by the beach. 'A little boy each and a girl together. That would be perfect.'

'Wouldn't it just,' Ian said.

I was full of optimism, and I had a good feeling about the future. Ian may not have been love's young dream, as Graham once was, but I was not a teenager any more. Ian was a good man, a dependable father and a loving husband. What more could I want? I honestly couldn't wish for anything else.

Chapter Eight

'Oh Christ, the head is coming out!'

'How long do you have to go?' the polite, softly-spoken GP asked me one night.

'This is my last shift,' I replied. 'I'm 29 weeks, just about.'

'Well, good luck,' he smiled. 'Make sure you have a good rest before the baby arrives.'

I promised I would. The GP was fairly new to the area and worked out of a practice in nearby Hyde. I'd seen him several times during my night shifts and he had a reputation for being extremely caring and always willing to join his patients at the hospital when they were in labour, even though he was not obliged to do so. I remember wishing there were more community-minded GPs like him.

I look back at that first encounter now and shudder. That GP was none other than Harold Shipman, who many years later would be identified as one of the most prolific serial killers in recorded history. I didn't know it then, but I would also become friendly with his wife Primrose outside of work, as our children attended the same village primary school during the Eighties.

That night I left him with his patient, who was labouring well and was several hours from giving birth. We midwives always welcomed an extra pair of professional hands on the labour ward, and it was comforting to be able to leave Dr Shipman looking after a patient for a while, freeing us up to check on other women who didn't have the luxury of having their GP turn up in the middle of the night.

In fact, we now know that Harold Shipman – or 'Fred' as we came to affectionately call him – was already a killer by this time, having claimed his first victim in 1975. I still can barely believe it to this day. He was admired by his patients and colleagues alike, and I never heard a single word said against him in all the years I knew him.

As it happened, this turned out to be a long and uneventful shift until the arrival of a woman called Belinda Vale, who came in shortly after 5 a.m. in what appeared to be the advanced stages of labour. Sister Norris asked me to examine her.

'Could you please remove your knickers?' I asked as Belinda heaved herself up onto a bed, breathing heavily and frowning with the pain. 'Then I can examine you and see how your labour is progressing.'

'No, thank you,' Belinda replied. She was a well-built, stern-faced lady, aged about thirty like me, and she clearly knew her own mind.

'Er, I just need you to take off your underwear …' I started.

'I'm not ready for that. I want to be here a little while before the baby comes. My mum won't be awake yet. If we give it a while she'll be able to catch the first bus at ten to seven.'

'I'm afraid the baby may not want to wait for your mum to arrive,' I explained. 'If the baby is ready to come out, you can't hold it back in.'

Belinda looked surprised and more than a little cross at this revelation. It has never failed to amaze me how very little some pregnant women know about the workings of the female body. Even today, when there is a plethora of pregnancy information available which wasn't accessible in the Seventies, I still encounter even the most well-educated of women who don't understand how the cervix opens, naturally, in preparation for the delivery.

'But I'm not ready,' Belinda began to protest hotly. A sharp contraction made her gasp in a mouthful of air. She exhaled huffily and said: 'Surely if I leave my knickers on that will hold the baby back in a bit longer …?'

I shook my head. 'I'm afraid not. You can't argue with Mother Nature. Once the contractions have started, the baby is getting ready to come out, and you can't change its mind.'

'Right,' Belinda said through pursed lips. 'Would you mind asking my husband to step in? I'd best get him to telephone my mum's neighbour so he can knock on her door and tell her what's going on.'

Belinda stoically delivered her baby without the use of pain relief or even gas and air just before I finished my shift at 7 a.m. She had a six-pound, seven-ounce baby girl she named Mandy, and as soon as she laid eyes on her daughter I swear Belinda's whole face changed. Her eyes were dewy, her deep frowns were replaced by laughter lines all around her mouth and eyelids, and even her voice softened. 'I like the Barry Manilow song, "Mandy",' she explained. 'I'm a bit soppy like that.'

I drove home with my head spinning. What a funny woman Belinda was. 'Soppy' was not a word I'd have used to describe her. Stubborn seemed more apt, but when a woman is in labour there is no telling which of her personality traits are going to spring to the fore. That's what I loved about my job, never really knowing what surprises were in store.

'Jonathan! Stuart! Can you come in for your tea?'

It was 22 June 1978 and I had made a spaghetti bolognese for the boys. Italian food was quite new to me, but I'd followed a recipe in my *Woman's Realm* magazine and Jonathan and Stuart loved it. They gobbled up a large plateful each in record time and dashed back outside to kick a ball around the garden, pretending they were star players for Manchester City or Manchester United.

I'd polished off a generous portion of pasta, too, and when I had a sudden pain in my stomach soon afterwards I fleetingly thought I had indigestion.

Moments later another, sharper pain rippled through my abdomen and I realised immediately that I was in labour. The contractions came on thick and fast and felt much more urgent than any labour pains I'd experienced when I'd had Jonathan. Now there was absolutely no danger of thinking I'd eaten too much, as I had done with the Christmas turkey, and I immediately telephoned my parents, who agreed to come over and take care of the boys. I then telephoned Ian's work.

'Hello, it's Linda Fairley, Ian Fairley's wife. Please can you give my husband a message?' I said very calmly.

Ian worked at Bootle Street police station in Manchester. It was impossible to phone him directly as he was normally out of the office, but I knew his colleague could radio him.

'Of course, love. What do I need to tell him?'

'Please tell him I'm in labour and please can he come home now.'

The desk policeman began to laugh. 'I can't believe how calm you are,' he said. 'I'll get the message to Ian straight away. Best of luck.'

Ian drove me to the hospital in his Austin Maxi, and he was very composed, too.

'Does it feel strange to have a baby where you work?' he asked.

'No, not really,' I replied. 'All the midwives I work with have their babies at Ashton. It's good to be in familiar surroundings.'

When we arrived at the Maternity Unit, Sister Kelly greeted me like a long-lost relative. 'It's good to see you, to be sure, Linda love. Is this your lovely husband? Graham, is it?'

Ian was unruffled by her mistake and didn't bother to protest. I'd been telling him recently that Sister Kelly had been getting a little forgetful, and he took her *faux pas* on the chin, like a real gentleman.

'Take yourself off to the labour ward, Linda love. I don't know who is on tonight.'

It was Anne Mortimer who greeted me on the labour ward. I knew Anne well and was pleased she would be taking care of me. We'd done some of our training together years before, although Anne had had to leave part way through to help out with her family business. She'd been back for a while now, and had earned herself an excellent reputation. Ian stayed by my side, too, and even though my contractions were excruciatingly painful I felt as comfortable as I could hope for.

Fiona was born at 10.30 p.m. after a labour lasting just three hours from the time I arrived on the labour ward. I had a shot of Pethidine in my buttock and I couldn't have cared less whether it was one of my colleagues or the Queen of Sheba giving me the jab. I needed the pain relief, and that was all that mattered. I had an episiotomy again, too, but I can barely recall it taking place.

'You're a model patient,' Anne flattered, although I know I cried and moaned and dug my fingers into Ian's hand many times, for which I later apologised.

'You're doing really well,' Ian told me throughout. 'I can't believe how restrained you are, actually.'

The labour was much easier than it had been with Jonathan, and I delivered Fiona really quite easily. I remember the feeling of euphoria much more than any feeling of pain.

Ian wasn't an overtly emotional man, but he looked deeply moved the first time he saw Fiona. She had extremely fine, downy white hair and a lovely round face. I didn't have to push for very long as, at seven pounds, eight ounces, she wasn't a big baby and was a good deal smaller than Jonathan. Fiona wasn't squashed or red-faced as some babies are. She was simply delightful, and she let out a shrill but somehow ladylike little cry, which brought a lump to my throat.

'We've got our little girl!' I whispered, a huge smile cracking across my face. I was too tired to speak any more, but lovely thoughts flitted through my head: 'One boy each, one beautiful daughter together. We're a perfect little family.'

Ian didn't want me to go back to work after my maternity leave with Fiona. We didn't need the money, as he was earning a good salary, but I was adamant I was returning to part-time nights. When I wasn't there, I missed everything about work. Just a few weeks after I had Fiona, the first test tube baby, Louise Brown, was born in Oldham General and District Hospital, which was less than five miles from Ashton General.

Sitting at home I watched the news being announced on the local BBC evening programme, North West Tonight, and my first thought was that I would have loved to discuss this important event with my colleagues. Louise was born on 25 July 1978 after being conceived in a test tube using an egg from her mother, Lesley, and sperm from her father, John. The newsreader explained that the resulting embryo was then placed back inside Lesley's body, where it developed in the normal way.

Excitement had been building up at Oldham for weeks as Louise's birth was imminent, and now there was jubilation that this miracle baby was healthy and normal, and had made medical history right on our doorstep.

'Isn't it great?' I said to my friend Sue when we chatted on the phone later that week. 'I can't believe it. I think it's such wonderful news.'

'It's amazing,' Sue replied. 'Though doesn't it make you realise how lucky we are to have had our children without having to go through anything like that?'

I had to agree. Sue now had Dylan as well as Miranda, and it really did feel that we were incredibly blessed to have both given birth to a son and a daughter each. It was always good to chat to Sue. Even after all these years, and despite the fact she lived many miles away in South Wales, the bond we'd first formed as seven-year-olds under the watchful eye of Sister Mary Francis at Harrytown High School had remained strong. In fact, having children had brought us even closer, and we always enjoyed swapping stories about raising our families.

'I am sure there are lots of women who might benefit from this,' Sue said.

'I'll say,' I replied excitedly. 'Honestly, this will change people's lives.'

Of course, in my job I did not deal directly with women who could not get pregnant at all, although I had met many who had suffered unexplained miscarriages. Back then, all we could do was cross our fingers and hope the poor lady managed to carry the next baby to full term, but all too often women suffered repeated miscarriages.

I returned to work in the spring of 1979, when Fiona was about ten months old and Margaret Thatcher had just become Britain's first female prime minister. I watched Maggie's victory speech on the ITV *News at Ten*. 'Where there is discord, may we bring harmony. Where there is error, may we bring truth. Where there is doubt, may we bring faith. And where there is despair, may we bring hope,' she said on the steps of Downing Street.

I hoped her policies would be good for the country, but most of all I admired her as a woman. 'Wow, there's a woman in Number 10!' was my very first reaction. That's what I said to Ian as we watched the victory speech together. I could scarcely believe it. It seemed only five minutes since women had been battling for equal pay; now, surely, we had true equality for the first time in history.

I was also pleased the country would have a fresh start after what had been a long winter of strikes. When the miners first went on strike in the so-called 'Winter of Discontent' in 1978, I supported them wholeheartedly and hoped their actions would help improve their pay and conditions, but as time went on I found it difficult to keep on being sympathetic. We had a lot of power cuts, and with Fiona being such a young baby at that time it made life very difficult for me whenever the lights and the heating and all my electric appliances went off. For example, I had an electric cooker, and so whenever the power went off I had to use a little Calor gas ring to warm the bottles. At night-time I had to do this by candlelight, which was really not much fun at all. I had not entertained the idea of breast-feeding this time round, after my bad experience with Jonathan, and I cursed my timing and bad luck at having to fiddle about with bottles in the cold and dark on winter nights.

Back at work, it was no surprise to find that many of my female colleagues shared my hopes about Margaret Thatcher giving us a great new start, and felt empowered to have a woman as prime minister.

'To be sure, Linda love,' Sister Kelly said when I passed her in the corridor on my first day back. 'That Maggie Thatcher's a fine example to us all.'

She nodded towards the TV lounge, where a newsreader was talking about the new Cabinet. The volume on the set was turned up very loud, but the half-dozen or so women listening and watching were all on the edge of their seats, clearly not wanting to miss a word.

Sister Kelly carried on down the corridor, passing a female doctor and saying, 'More power to your elbow' to her as she did so.

'Excuse me?' the doctor said.

'I were just sayin',' I heard Sister Kelly explain. 'Maggie Thatcher. What a victory for us women, eh?'

The doctor smiled and said, 'Yes, but she will have to be *better* than a man to succeed.'

'There speaks a woman of experience,' Sister Kelly snorted as she went on her way. In typical style she retrieved her underwear from between her buttocks as she walked off. In spite of her eccentricities, I couldn't agree more with Sister Kelly's sentiment, or that of the female doctor. Maggie Thatcher had set the bar high, and now we women had to prove ourselves more than ever.

The phone rang at the nurses' station on the labour ward just as I was settling into my very first shift back.

'Please help,' a breathless man implored. 'I think the baby is coming.'

I had never helped to deliver a baby down the telephone before, but I knew the drill. It was a scenario that was becoming more common in the late Seventies, as more people had a home telephone. Knowing they could call from the house at any time of the day or night, without the uncertainty of having to knock up a neighbour or run to a telephone box, seemed to have given people the confidence to hold on just that bit longer, and occasionally just that bit too long.

'What is happening?'

'My wife is in labour and I think I can see the baby's head!'

'Right, stay on the phone and please …'

'We need an ambulance!'

'We will get one to you as soon as possible. Stay on the phone and please give me your wife's name and your address quickly, and then tell me what is happening.'

'Oh Christ, the head is coming out!'

'That's OK. Please tell me your name and …'

'Potter. Jean Potter, 22 Mile Lane.'

My colleague Stella grabbed the piece of paper I'd written the name on and immediately picked up another phone to call the ambulance service, using a direct line we had to the depot. She would also dispatch a community midwife to the address.

'Right, the ambulance will be with you very soon.'

'Thank Christ!'

'Mr Potter, don't hang up, but please can you go to your wife and tell her not to push hard. Little pushes are good. And have you got a towel to hand?'

'A towel? Love, have we got a towel?'

I could hear poor Mrs Potter grunting and crying.

'Don't worry if you haven't got a towel. Use anything you have to hand in the room that you can use to wrap the baby up in. Please don't leave your wife.'

'OK. There's my dressing gown on the back of the door. Shall I go and get it?'

'That's good. Put the phone down for a minute but don't hang up. Come back to me when you have got the dressing gown.'

I heard him tell his wife, rather unconvincingly, that he knew what he was doing. His voice quaked.

'Nurse! Are you still there?! The baby's head is out and it's starting to cry! It's body is still inside, though!'

'That's good, the baby's body will come in a minute or two. Is your wife in a safe place to deliver the rest of the baby?'

'Yes, she's on the bed. The baby's out now!'

'That's good. Is the baby pink?'

'Oh, yes.'

'That's good. I can hear it crying. Well done. Wrap the baby up with the dressing gown but leave it between your wife's legs.'

He put the receiver down again and did as he was told without questioning me. I didn't want him to pick up the baby, in case the cord was short and he might snap it. I didn't explain this, as there wasn't time and I didn't want to alarm him.

'I'm back.'

'What's happening now? Is the baby warm?'

'Yes, the baby's warm and – that's the doorbell!'

'That's good. Go and let them in, then come straight back and please put the ambulanceman on the phone to me.'

Moments later an ambulanceman came on the line and confirmed that the baby was out and seemed fine. I reassured him a community midwife had been dispatched to the address and would be there very soon.

'Can I have a word?" I head Mr Potter ask in the background.

'Hello? Are you still there, Nurse?'

'I am. Congratulations, Mr Potter.'

'Thank you, Nurse. Thank you very much. I couldn't have done it without you.'

'I'm glad I could help, but you were the one who was there. Well done. You should be very proud. Please pass on my congratulations to your wife.'

'I will!' he replied. The excitement in his voice was palpable, and I wished I were there to share in the joy.

When the call ended I felt slightly flat, actually. I wanted to hold on to that new life that had just emerged, to wrap the baby up and see the look of triumph and satisfaction on the mother's face. As it was I didn't even know if it was a boy or a girl!

Still, I was very pleased that the birth had run so smoothly. In years to come as I did more 'telephone deliveries', I would learn that this was quite typical of what happens in such circumstances.

Generally speaking, it is not usually a first baby when the delivery is so rapid, and so the woman has a good idea what she is doing. In addition, as she has received no sedation and there has been no delay in the delivery, there's a jolly good chance the baby will breathe immediately.

I had been taught that if the baby didn't cry in such cases you would have to say to the father, 'Quickly, rub the baby and blow on its face and chest, to stimulate it.' If the baby's face was going blue during the delivery, you would have to ask the husband to check if the cord was round the baby's neck, and to loosen it if possible. Thankfully, I have never had to give such instructions, and in every such case I have dealt with, the birth has ended with the father feeling like an absolute hero at having assisted in delivering his own child.

Mrs Potter would be visited by the community midwife for the next ten days, and she would probably need to unload a little more than most women about the birth, as she would no doubt be shocked at the speed of the delivery. The community midwife would reassure her that she had done a great job, and encourage her to talk about how she felt, to help her recover.

As I was leaving the hospital the next morning after my night shift, I bumped into Mrs Tattersall in the car park. Even though almost a decade had passed since I'd first met her when I was a pupil midwife in 1970, Mrs Tattersall looked exactly the same as she always did. Dragging on a cigarette, she was hauling a bag of instruments into the boot of her car. She'd swapped her green Avenger for a Rover several years before, but this vehicle looked just as dirty and unloved as her old one.

'Linda! How are ya keepin', love?' she asked briskly.

'Really well,' I replied. 'I'm not long back from maternity leave. I've got a little girl now, too.'

'So I heard,' Mrs Tattersall replied, reminding me that there wasn't much that happened at the hospital, or indeed in its vicinity, that Mrs Tattersall didn't know about. 'Well done, love. And happily remarried too, I hear. Well done.'

'Thanks. How have you been?'

'Same as ever,' she tutted. 'Run ragged, ruddy babies poppin' out here, there and everywhere. Can't stop. Poor lass in Mottram locked herself out of the house. Ended up having the baby in her neighbour's bed, would you believe.'

I wanted to tell Mrs Tattersall about my telephone delivery, and wished I could ask her about all the other interesting encounters she had no doubt had, but of course she was in a tearing hurry, as always.

'Good to see you looking so well. Bye, love,' she called over her shoulder as she got in her car and turned on the engine. It didn't start first time and I saw her cursing under her breath and rolling her eyes before finally driving away, black clouds of smoke belching out of the Rover's noisy exhaust pipe. Good old Mrs Tattersall, I thought. I'd loved my time with her out in the community, and in that moment I realised I'd like to get back out there one day, when the time was right.

Chapter Nine

'The bigger the medallion,
the harder they fall'

Janet Cresswell arrived on the ward minutes after I arrived for a shift one evening in November 1979. She was clutching her stomach but didn't appear to be in labour.

'Hope I'm not wasting your time,' she said. 'But I've got terrible pains in my stomach. My husband says it's probably that fish supper I had for me tea, but I thought it better to be safe than sorry!'

She had a bubbly, infectious laugh and a very engaging way of talking. Her eyes fell on my MRI bronze penny, which I always pinned proudly on my uniform. 'Well, I never!' Janet remarked. 'Did you train at the MRI?'

'Yes,' I replied proudly. 'That's very observant of you.'

'Not really,' Janet replied. 'I worked there myself for a year, in the kitchens back in 1969.'

'Well, I never. That's when I was there. What a small world it is. I used to love afternoon tea the best. We used to race to get there for the lovely warm bread, and we'd pile on thick butter and loads of strawberry jam …'

I showed Janet into the admissions room. She had her sister Joyce with her, who settled on a chair beside the bed while Janet lay down and waited to be examined. Stella was the other midwife on duty, and she stepped into the room to check

Janet's blood pressure. I could hear the three women chatting and giggling as I returned to the desk to collect the notes for another patient I had been assigned to look after in a labour room.

'I'm not buying me supper from that chippie ever again,' I heard Janet chuckle.

'Could have just been the mushy peas,' her sister joked. 'Or maybe it was that doorstep of bread and butter you wolfed down, too!'

'I'm allowed now I'm eating for two ...'

I had been allocated to care for a lovely Irish lady called Rita Barrow. Rita was known to many of the midwives as she had delivered six babies in the unit over the previous seven years, including a set of twins. I had never actually delivered her before and I felt quite pleased to finally have the chance to join the large band of midwives who had contributed to bringing Rita's considerable brood into the world.

'You're new!' Rita exclaimed when she saw me.

'Not really, I've been here since the unit opened. I've been off on maternity leave twice, though. Perhaps that's why we haven't met.'

'You might be right,' Rita said. 'Or do you always work nights? I normally have my babies during the daytime. Maybe I'll hang on until the morning, ya never know.'

After examining Rita I told her that looked unlikely. Her labour was well established and, even though she didn't appear to be in the advanced stages, I estimated she only had two or three hours to go.

She settled into a steady routine of grumbling through her contractions, cursing the Catholic church for making her forgo contraception, and reminiscing about the birth of little Jimmy

– or was it Patrick, Rory or Kieran? – she couldn't be sure. Her twins were girls, delivered naturally four years earlier. Rita had only had gas and air and didn't tear during the twins' birth, she reminded me proudly, several times.

From time to time Rita picked up an old magazine from her bag and flicked though for a story to comment on. 'Look at dem punks,' she scoffed, showing me pictures of young people with pink Mohican haircuts. 'If any o' mine turned out like that I'd have their guts for garters, so I would. Ow. Owwwww. Urgh. How long d'you reckon, Nurse?'

Rita's labour was unexpectedly slow and gradual, even stop-start at times. This gave her ample time to chat about all manner of topics. Margaret Thatcher was one. 'It's about time a woman got a shot at the top job,' Rita declared, echoing what so many women were saying. 'Show those men how to do it, so she can. And put a stop to all the doom and gloom the socialists have caused.'

I didn't have any strong political views, but I had to agree that the country did seem to have been in a miserable state for a lot of the Seventies. When I thought back to the Sixties, I wondered what had happened to all the fun and all the talk of peace and love and flower-power I thought would last forever. It had been replaced by industrial unrest and anarchy, and what's more, instead of my beloved Beatles belting out pop music on the radio, we had glam rock stars like Gary Glitter and the tartan-clad Bay City Rollers taking over the hit parade, both of whom I think I must have been too old to appreciate.

'Roll on the Eighties!' Rita said at one point, and I found myself agreeing with her. The Seventies had seen me grow from a newly qualified young midwife into a confident mother of two. I was more competent at my job than ever before and was settled in my family life with Ian, but I'd had tough times, too.

Breaking up with Graham had not been easy, and looking back it had taken me a good while to really get back on my feet, despite being with Ian. Things were much better now. Graham still saw Jonathan regularly, of course, and we had an amicable relationship after a time of change and unrest. Things could only get better, I was sure.

Rita finally delivered at 3 a.m. Her husband had stayed at home with the other children and I remained at Rita's bedside the whole time, as the unit was extremely busy and there was nobody to relieve me, even for a short break.

The baby was huge – a ten-pound, nine-ounce boy who needed a full hour of pushing for Rita to deliver. She was absolutely exhausted afterwards, and quite indignant, too.

'How can that be?' she asked. 'How can a seventh child be so hard to deliver?'

'It's just the position he was in,' I replied. 'He's such a big baby, he was never going to come out that easily, despite all the others before him.'

Rita held her new baby boy tight and started to tell him all the names of his brothers and sisters. She was that tired she could barely speak, but I could see the love in her eyes. I congratulated her warmly, and when an auxiliary finally came in to help me tidy up I slipped out for a much-needed break.

It was eerily quiet on the corridor for what I knew to be a busy shift. I went to the office and found Stella in floods of tears. Barbara Lees had her arms around her and I realised Barbara was crying, too. 'What on earth's happened?' I asked nervously.

They both tried to talk but broke down again. A red-eyed Sister Norris appeared in the doorway behind me, told me to sit down and proceeded to tell me very solemnly what had gone on while I'd been occupied with Rita, on the other side of the labour ward.

Janet Cresswell, unbelievably, had died. 'We are all struggling to take it in,' Sister Norris said. Her words winded me, or at least that's how it felt. I gasped for breath as she proceeded to tell me how this had happened to such a vibrant, apparently healthy young woman.

I learned that when Stella had checked Janet's blood pressure it was sky high. Janet also had some oedema, or swelling, around her ankles, and there was protein in her urine. I knew before Sister Norris said the word 'pre-eclampsia' that this was what she was talking about. As a pupil midwife I had been trained meticulously in this condition and, as with every midwife, its symptoms were constantly at the forefront of my mind. It is one of the main reasons midwives always monitor blood pressure and check for protein in the urine.

We also routinely check for oedema, although on its own this is not usually a problem. However, oedema and raised blood pressure set off an alarm bell, telling the midwife to keep a close eye on this patient. If there is protein in the urine in addition to swelling and raised blood pressure, it may become an emergency situation. We don't know why it happens, but the raised levels of protein irritate the brain, and can cause an eclamptic fit. Tragically, this is what had happened to Janet.

'She was laughing and joking one minute and then she suddenly started to fit,' I heard Sister Norris say, though the words were so awful, so unbelievable, I was struggling to take them in. It was as if I had walked into a dark cloud and my senses were obscured, though I felt hot tears streaming down my cheeks.

'And she fitted and fitted and fitted, continuously. We did everything …' Sister Norris began to cry, too, and through her tears she told me that Janet was held down and then sedated as quickly as possible to contain the fit, as was the correct procedure. An eclamptic fit is not like an epileptic fit that might last for a matter of minutes. This type can go on and on and on. Nowadays, if a patient presents in such a way they are not only sedated but also given a powerful cocktail of drugs to bring down their high blood pressure.

Catastrophically for Janet, we didn't have the drugs or the knowledge to do this back in 1979, and despite rushing her to theatre and getting her sedated as quickly as possible, she lost her life. She was thirty-two weeks pregnant, twenty-nine years old and the mother of a four-year-old boy.

I don't remember driving home early that morning after my shift ended at 7 a.m.; I just remember holding my own children extra tight and counting my blessings over and over again. I learned the following week that Janet's husband had been heartbreakingly kind, telling my colleagues he knew they had tried so very hard to save her. He had also asked Stella, 'How can I tell my little boy he has lost his mummy and the new baby?' which triggered another flood of tears.

Several of my colleagues went to the funeral and stayed in touch with Janet's husband for many months afterwards. It was very important to the midwives to know that he accepted this support, and he had reassured all the staff that he understood there was nothing more that could have been done to save his wife. Nevertheless, it was a devastating event for the whole maternity unit.

I thought about Janet every day for a very long time. It was only a matter of weeks before Christmas, and I remember shopping for presents and decorating my home and thinking how awful it must be for Janet's husband, trying to carry on and make things special for his son. I felt a pang of guilt on many occasions when I shared a joke with Ian or enjoyed watching Fiona make her brothers giggle. They absolutely adored her, and she had really cemented our family together. It didn't seem fair that I had so much and Janet had lost everything.

On New Year's Eve 1979 Ian took me to a police dinner dance in Manchester while my parents babysat for us. We did the same thing each New Year and, to be honest, I wasn't particularly excited about it. I never felt I had much in common with Ian's police friends, although they were always very welcoming and their wives were usually good company. Anyhow, I bought myself a long black evening dress that crossed over at the back, and I really made an effort to look my best, telling myself that we'd have a good evening, and that I should make the most of it.

In fact, it turned out to be a fantastic night. As it was not only New Year's Eve but the end of the decade, it seemed that everybody had really pushed the boat out. The meal was roast lamb with all the trimmings, which was delicious, the hotel function room sparkled with wonderful decorations and all the guests looked terrific, with the men in tuxedos and the women in beautiful long dresses and glittery stilettos. The atmosphere was electric, and I remember a lot of excited talk about the start of the new decade.

I had great fun dancing at the disco after the meal. Blondie's 'Heart of Glass' was playing when I first got up with a group of women. We left the men sitting around drinking pints, smoking cigars and looking after our little sequinned evening bags, which we left on the table. Gloria Gaynor's 'I Will Survive' got us all singing in unison as we danced in a circle, and I felt filled with optimism. Ian planted a big kiss on my lips as the clock struck midnight.

'Here's to the Eighties!' I said. 'Happy New Year!' All felt well with the world, and as we travelled home in a taxi I counted my blessings.

Looking back now, the Eighties always make me think of medallion men, and women with big shoulder pads. It was the era when women were starting to really believe they could have it all. For the first time in my experience, women were starting to return to work within a matter of weeks of giving birth. They wanted to prove they could pop out babies one minute and return to the office wearing killer heels and power suits the next.

I think having a female prime minister had something to do with it as, whatever one thought of her politics, Margaret Thatcher seemed to make women from many different walks of life feel more empowered than they had done in the Seventies.

The case of Monica Duggan and her husband Chris is the first one that comes to mind whenever I think of this era.

'I hope this isn't a false alarm,' I heard Monica complain through the curtain that was pulled around her bed one evening in November 1980. 'I really don't want to be sent home.'

Monica was bending her husband's ear as she laboured in the first-stage room, and I'd been sent to examine her.

'It's the midwife here,' I called through the floral fabric, which was faded and worn and badly in need of replacing. 'Can I come in?'

'Yes, please do,' Monica replied. 'I'm hoping you can get things moving a bit quicker than they are.'

Her husband pulled a face in mock horror. 'What are you like?' he smirked, looking slightly embarrassed. 'You're not on a deadline now, you know.'

'I know, I know. But you have to admit it would be good to have this baby tonight. It wouldn't half help.'

I discovered that Monica worked in advertising and held a senior position in a well-known company. She had gone into labour two weeks before her due date, and as she wanted to return to work as soon as possible, having her baby early would reduce the length of time she would be taking off for maternity leave. She reminded her husband of this impatiently, telling him it would help prove she could juggle the job and the baby, which would 'show that Roger in personnel' what she was capable of.

Monica certainly looked like a businesswoman to be reckoned with. Her blonde hair was immaculately styled and a strong smell of hairspray emanated from her head. She wore bright red lipstick and had come straight from work in the centre of Manchester, where she had experienced her first labour pains as she 'wrapped up a presentation' at 8 p.m. She was wearing a scarlet suit to match her lipstick, the jacket of which had the biggest shoulder pads I had ever seen, and a short skirt that was pulled halfway up her bump and was partially covered with a billowing cream silk blouse. To complete the outfit she wore a pair of black kitten heels with fancy gold buckles across the front.

'Shall we get you more comfortable?' I suggested, offering to help her out of the jacket and shoes. 'And I think in order to examine you we might need to get you out of that little skirt …'

Monica obliged rather begrudgingly, and I was able to establish that she was in fact only two centimetres dilated and had many more hours of labour ahead of her yet. She complained at length and asked again if there was anything I could do to speed things up.

When I told her that no, we should wait for nature to take its course, she sent Chris home with a very specific list of items to collect. He was to fetch her Sony Walkman, her Blondie cassette tape, her new copy of *Company* magazine and a business brochure she had promised a colleague she would look over.

'Can I have a bath?' Monica asked me impatiently. 'To help with the pain?'

'Yes, though I'd wait until Chris is back and he can help you, and you might get more benefit from it if you wait a while.'

'Fine,' she agreed, and I promised to pop back later to check everything was as it should be.

It was perhaps inevitable that Monica's birth did not go entirely according to plan. I've seen on many occasions that when a woman tries to be too controlling she is likely to make herself stressed, when what you really need before a delivery is for the woman to relax as much as possible.

When Monica finally took her bath in the early hours of the morning she was in quite a strop, as her labour had progressed very slowly. Chris accompanied her to the door of the bathroom and sat outside obediently after filling the bath to the specified height and temperature demanded by Monica.

I noticed he had changed out of his shiny business suit when he nipped home and was now wearing a sort of new-age white shirt with a ruffle down the front. It looked like something one of the Bee Gees might wear, and he'd teamed it with extremely tight jeans that were held up with a flash, studded belt. Chris had a hairy chest, which was very visible as he had at least the top three buttons of his shirt undone, and I saw that he was wearing a heavy gold medallion around his neck.

'How are you doing?' I asked him.

'Everything's under control,' he said coolly. 'I know how to handle Monica. Don't worry. She'll be fine. The bath will help her chill out.'

'That's good,' I replied. 'Let's hope so.'

Ten minutes later Chris came running down the corridor, shouting and screaming.

'Help! Come quick! Monica's still in the bath and the baby's coming.' He had completely lost his cool and began tugging on my sleeve like a little lost boy.

'Don't panic,' I said, grabbing a delivery pack. 'I'm here. She'll be fine. Come on. Take a deep breath and come with me.'

I found Monica in an even more distraught state than Chris. She had pulled the plug out of the bath in a panic when her contractions suddenly intensified and she thought she felt the urge to push, but then had been unable to lift herself out of the deep tub. That's when she yelled for Chris to help, and he had charged off to find me.

By the time I arrived in the bathroom Monica was naked and shivering with cold in the empty bath, screaming blue murder. Her red lipstick was smudged around her lips and her hair was sticking out in all directions, making her look quite a fright.

'Don't worry,' I said. 'We'll get you out and everything will be absolutely fine.'

I packed Chris off to fetch more towels from the linen cupboard just across the corridor and asked Monica if she felt able to lift herself out of the bath, with my help.

'Of course I bloody well can't!' she screamed. 'Do you think I'd be sitting here if I could?! Aaaarrrggghhhhh!'

She flung her head back dramatically when the contraction tightened across her abdomen, banging the back of her head on the taps. Then she began to cry, her tears depositing clumps of mascara around her eyes. When Chris returned moments later, he and I had quite a job lifting Monica out of the bath, as she did nothing to help us.

'I can't, I can't,' she wailed as she sat there covered in goose bumps.

'You can, you can,' we assured her, finally hauling her cumbersome body out of the bath.

It was three more hours before Monica finally gave birth in the labour ward. She continued to be an extremely difficult patient throughout, moaning and cursing through every contraction, and snapping at Chris and me in turn.

'These sheets are like cardboard!' she complained. 'Get me a bloody drink, Chris, I'm parched.'

Later, she grumbled several times: 'That gas and air is worse than useless!'

My head was banging when the baby finally arrived, but not nearly as much as Chris's head was.

'Where is he?' Monica asked as I placed her seven-pound, four-ounce daughter in her arms at just before 5 a.m. and she looked up to share the proud moment with her husband.

'Chris?' I said. 'I'm ever so sorry but he's on the floor. He's fainted, I'm afraid. He's going to need a couple of stitches in his head. He'll be with you shortly.'

Chris had keeled over at the precise moment his daughter was born, banging his head on the corner of a trolley. I'd buzzed for assistance and a nurse had rushed in to attend to him. Monica had been so focused on giving birth she had not even noticed.

'He'll need more than a *couple* of stitches, but he'll be fine,' the nurse whispered to me. 'He must have come quite a cropper.'

'Did he? I think it's a case of the bigger the medallion, the harder they fall,' I replied cheekily.

I hadn't intended Monica to overhear that remark, but she did and it made her giggle, even though Chris was now coming round and it was his turn to moan in pain. Monica was rocking her baby tenderly in her arms, and her laughing eyes were filled with love. 'What a beauty you are,' she said to her baby girl. 'What an absolute beauty you are.'

We all know that childbirth is a life-changing event, but looking at Monica that day I really hoped that it might change her life more than most. Later, when I nipped up to the post-natal ward after I finished my shift, to my delight I found Monica and Chris peering lovingly at baby Charlene in her cot. She really was a pretty little girl and I felt a tear come into my eye when I saw that Chris had been crying.

He and Monica looked like completely different people to the two I'd first met the night before. They were mellow and relaxed and looked full of love rather than ambition and rivalry. Chris was sporting a large gauze plaster on the back of his head but he didn't seem bothered one bit about that, and there was no mention from Monica about work, or how she'd had her wish and given birth before her due date. I wished them well and went home feeling emotionally drained, but happy.

I considered how fortunate I was to be doing the job I adored without having to have sharp elbows under a power suit, as I imagined businesswomen like Monica did. I didn't want promotion and I was not interested in rising up the ranks at Tameside or moving to another hospital to take on a more senior position. What's more, I could fit my work very well around my family.

I didn't judge women like Monica, but they did make me realise how lucky I was to have found satisfaction in a job that was so very real. Thinking of the way Monica looked as she cradled her baby, I was sure she'd find a good balance in her life, too. I really hoped so.

I met many more women like Monica throughout the Eighties and they always made me cherish my own children even more, if that were possible. 'Work is not as important as your children,' I wished I could say to them when they stressed about calling the office or talking to their boss when they were in labour.

'Enjoy this time, you can't get it back,' I sometimes wished I could tell them. I knew they would discover this in their own good time, however, and it certainly wasn't my place to give these women my opinion.

I really *did* prize the time I spent with my own children, watching them grow up. Ian was always full of good ideas, surprising us with a trip on a submarine on one memorable occasion, or taking the boys to watch Manchester United (despite the fact Jonathan insisted he was a City fan like Graham!) while I took Fiona to the park.

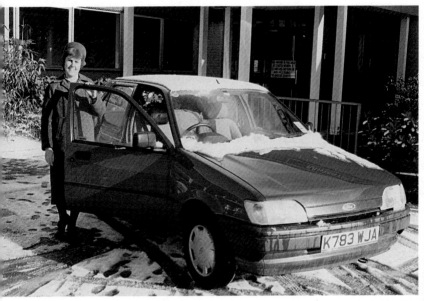

Outside Tameside Maternity Unit, winter 1991. I was on my way to visit a mother and baby I'd delivered a few days earlier. Fortunately, it wasn't as dramatic as Sarah Heywood's delivery, when I had to abandon my car in the snow!

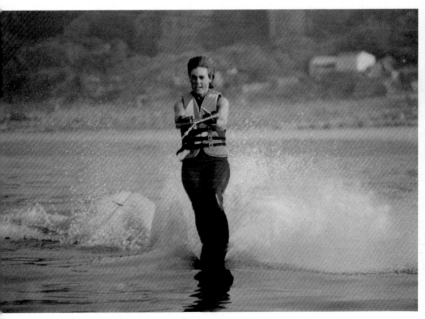

Water-skiing in Anglesey: I'd swapped my uniform for a wetsuit.

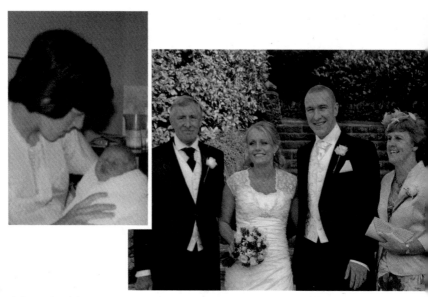

The midwife becomes a mother! Here with two-day-old Fiona in 1978 – lying in the room that was normally my workplace, marvelling at this new life that was now such a huge responsibility to me, was absolutely mind-blowing. Both of my children have made me so proud, particularly when my late husband Peter (*far left*) and I watched Fiona marry her Prince Charming, Pete (*centre*), in 2010.

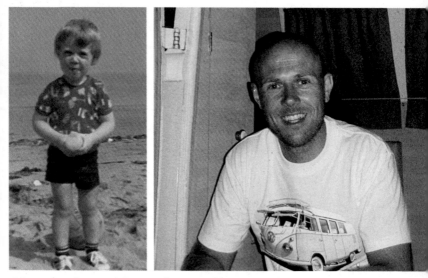

My son Jonathan aged three, and now aged 38. It's amazing how fast time flies – it feels like only yesterday that I thought I'd eaten too many turkey sandwiches when I had in fact gone into labour with him!

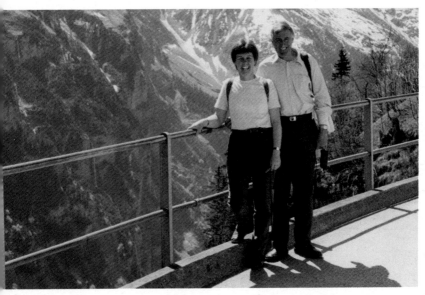

Peter and me on our honeymoon in Switzerland. I was so lucky to have another chance of love, even if it was too brief. I wish he could have been here to see this book published; I've cherished every moment as Peter would have wanted.

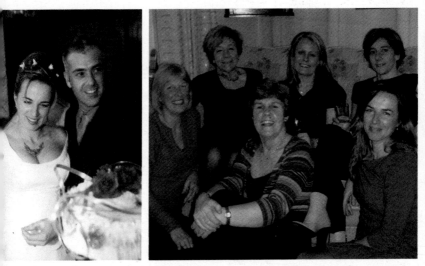

My nephew Kerem and his beautiful wife Elida on their wedding day in December 2000 (*above left*). Tragically, it was only three months later that Kerem was killed in Kosovo; it breaks my heart that he never got to meet his daughter Tara. We're a strong family and we got through it together – here I'm with Nevim, Fiona, Tijen, Elida and my friend Chris (*clockwise from top left*).

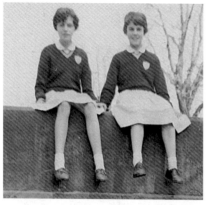

Here come the girls!

Top: Me, aged 14, with school friend Sue Smith (*left*).

Middle: This time we're all aged 40, with Angela (*far left*), Sue Smith (*second left*) and Sue Thornley (*second right*).

Bottom: The same gang aged 60! Sue Thornley is standing on the left, followed by Angela, Sue Smith, my mum and me. Nothing has changed over the years – apart from a few more wrinkles, I guess!

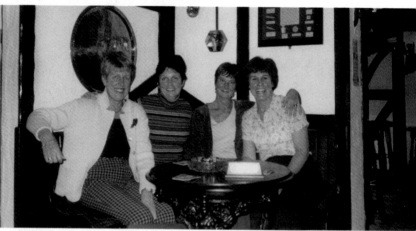

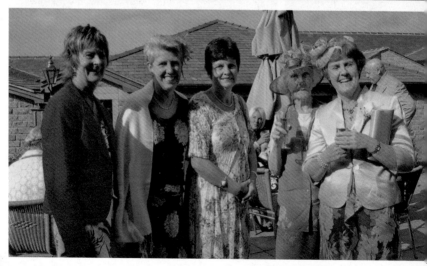

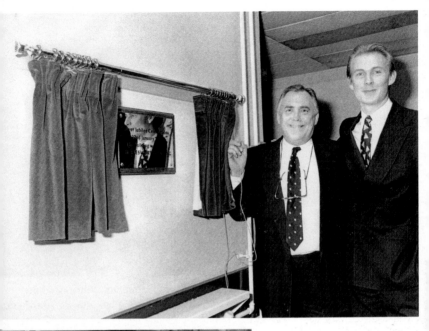

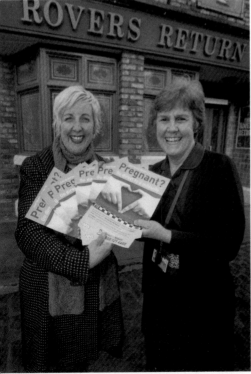

Above: *Coronation Street* star Bill Tarmey, who played Jack Duckworth, and Jarrod Randle, who was the first baby to be born at the new maternity unit at Tameside, helping us to celebrate its 25th anniversary. You would have thought that with *Coronation Street* being such a popular show, particularly in Manchester, I would have recognised actress Julie Hesmondhalgh, who played Hayley Cropper, when she came into my clinic! Fortunately, she wasn't offended and has since generously supported the Manchester midwifery community, even inviting a number of local midwives on to the set of *Coronation Street* (*left*).

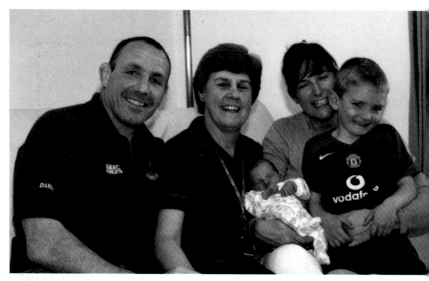

With my dear friend and colleague Helen, her husband Dean, son William and my goddaughter Anna, whom I'd delivered a few days earlier. I felt very honoured to have been at the heart of such a wonderful event in my friend's life. I often get asked to be a godmother to babies I have delivered, but it's a big commitment and not a role I take on lightly. I want to make sure I do the job properly, so I have only four godchildren in total.

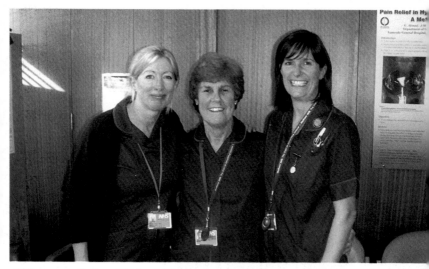

With Angela (*left*) and Helen (*right*) at my retirement party in 2008. It was a wonderful day, and everyone made me feel very special, but I sensed even then that I was not going to accept my days of being a midwife were over. True enough, three weeks later I was back in work – and I'm still happily delivering babies to this day!

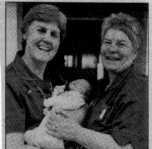

THE ADVERTISER, THURSDAY, MAY 5, 2011

SHORTLISTED... Linda Fairley (left) and Julie Evans

Midwives are in line for national awards

TWO midwives who have clocked up more than 70 years delivering babies have been shortlisted for national awards.

Julie Evans and Linda Fairley, who both work at Tameside hospital, have been shortlisted for midwife and community midwife of the year respectively in the British Journal of Midwifery Practice awards.

Julie was nominated for her work with two women who suffered stillbirths 30 years ago.

Linda, who is the UK's longest-serving midwife at a single hospital, is hoping to add another trophy to her collection after recently being named Cheshire woman of the year.

She said: "Just to be in the running for this award is fantastic, especially at the end of my career. It would be very special if I won."

Julie and Linda will find out tonight if they have won the awards during a ceremony in Manchester.

2669. www.tamesidereporter.com   17

What an honour

NOMINATION: Linda Fairley.

A LONG-SERVING Tameside Hospital midwife is celebrating after being shortlisted for the prestigious Cheshire Woman of the Year Award.

Linda Fairley, from Mottram, has been nominated in the Professional Success and Community Service categories, having served for 42 years as a midwife at the hospital before retiring.

She has now been invited, along with other nominees from across Cheshire and the Wirral, to attend a special celebratory lunch, where their personal courage, ourstanding professional success or services to their community will be celebrated.

The worthy winner will be presented with an engraved silver salver and a cheque to give to her chosen charity, as part of the lunch at Eaton Park, on April 6.

The Cheshire Woman of the Year award has been recognising worthy women since 1984 and has raised more than £200,000 to help children in Cheshire and Wirral.

Last year the awards raised over £7,000 for the NSPCC.

Money raised this year will support the charity's vital helpline services, ChildLine and the NSPCC helpline.

Anyone interested in supporting the NSPCC, or for more information about fundraising, can contact the North West Appeals Team on (0161) 628 1209 or email northwestappeals@nspcc.org.uk

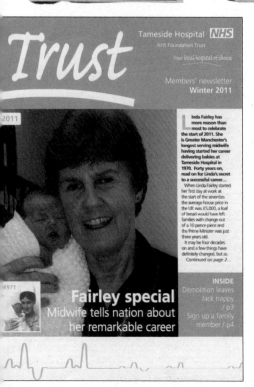

Top left and right: I was so honoured to receive a Lifetime Achievement Award at the Cheshire Woman of the Year awards, and also to be nominated as a Community Midwife of the Year by the *British Journal of Midwifery*. Sadly, Peter died before the award ceremonies, but I can still hear his voice saying, 'You can do it!' That's why I've dedicated this book to him.

Left: 'The oldest midwife in the world!' The front page of the Tameside Hospital newsletter, which started the amazing chain of events that led to me writing my books.

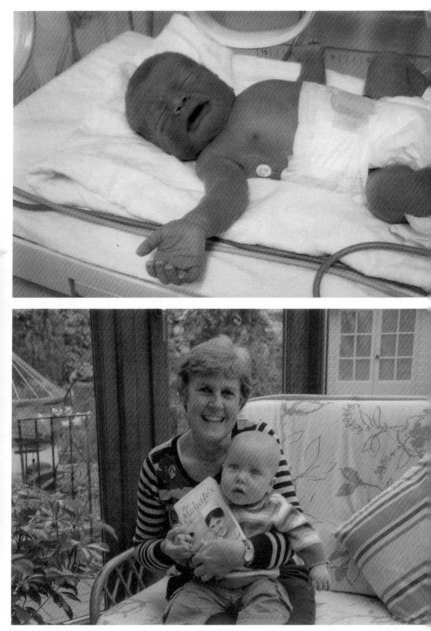

Top: My grandson Joel, aged just 20 minutes, in an incubator. He arrived five weeks early and was a little miracle. *Above*: Joel and me on the day I received a copy of my first book, *The Midwife's Here!*

We didn't have lots of extravagant holidays or expensive treats, as many children do nowadays, but we had plenty of fun. When Charles and Diana got married in 1981, for instance, we were staying in a caravan in Anglesey. We decorated the van with flags and there was a children's party on the campsite. Jonathan and Stuart had an absolute ball drinking orange squash out of plastic cups with Union Jacks on them and playing musical statues. Fiona was only three and she amused herself by climbing up and down the caravan steps over and over again. She drove me mad with it, but I couldn't be cross with her. I can still see her cheeky little face and blonde curls. She could get away with anything.

Most summers I volunteered to help run the first aid tent at the Mottram C of E Primary School fair, where Fiona and Jonathan were pupils. Harold Shipman, the friendly local GP I knew simply as Fred back then, usually helped me. He wore a Red Cross uniform and looked very smart in a pressed white shirt with epaulettes on the shoulders. Between us we hauled out trestle tables and set up the stall, and we spent several hours taking it in turns to man the stand, or sitting there together and chatting in between dishing out plasters for cut knees and antiseptic cream for grazed elbows.

'Isn't it funny how it's always the same people who tip up to help?' I said to Fred on a balmy Saturday in July 1983. We were batting away wasps that were attracted to a dollop of ice cream a child had dropped on the grass near our stand.

'I know,' he replied. 'These types of thing certainly show who has community spirit.'

The day before the fair I'd popped to Fred's home to deliver a batch of biscuits to Primrose, who was helping to run the cake stall. We had a cup of tea together in the kitchen and chatted about our children.

'How's Fiona settling into the school?' Primrose asked.

'She's loving it,' I replied. 'Jonathan's always been very happy there, and I didn't have any worries about Fiona settling in. She's a very sociable little girl.'

Primrose talked about the different personalities of her four children, two of whom were older than Jonathan and Fiona. One was close in age to Fiona at that time, and the youngest was still a toddler. Primrose clearly doted on them all, and enjoyed telling me about their different characters.

'Jonathan has always been a quiet little boy,' I told her in return. 'When he was younger he used to play very gently with his Lego and farm animals, but Fiona's the opposite and never stops talking and buzzing around. She's full of confidence, chatting on about her dollies and never giving her brothers a minute's peace!'

'That's girls for you,' Primrose commented as she beat her cake mixture in a ceramic bowl.

I relayed a story that has become one of our family favourites; so much so that Jonathan actually told it at Fiona's wedding in 2009. I'd taken the children to see *The Sooty Show* in Manchester and Fiona was sick all over her clothes. In typical flamboyant style, she took off her dress and sat through the show in her knickers and vest rather than miss out, while Jonathan was so mortified he couldn't even watch the rest of the performance.

'Mind you, I suppose he is almost five years older,' I conceded, and Primrose and I both laughed about it as I drained my teacup and we said our goodbyes.

When I look back now I really cannot believe that I was in Harold Shipman's home, drinking tea with his wife, and then running a first aid tent with Shipman himself in such a civilised, ordinary manner. It makes me feel ill to think of it.

The following year, not long after the summer fair, Fiona fell and cut her face on a piece of furniture at home. It was quite a nasty cut and I took her to A&E, which was absolutely heaving. A nurse put three small stitches in the wound, but on the way home I made a snap decision to call in at Harold Shipman's. I was afraid Fiona might end up with a scar on her face and just wanted a second opinion and some friendly advice from a doctor I trusted, and whom I considered to be a family friend. He gently removed the stitches and put three disposable butterfly sutures over the wound instead.

'There, there,' he soothed as Fiona winced. 'That should do the job. I think that will heal up without leaving a scar.'

He gave me a reassuring smile and I felt so much better. I can hardly bring myself to say it, but he honestly had what appeared to be a very genuine concern for his patients. On that day he instantly tuned in to my maternal concerns, replacing the stitches without question, even though the work of the A&E nurse was probably perfectly adequate. He did it for me, because he could see I was worried and that removing the stitches would make me feel better, and I was very grateful to him. Again, I look back at that encounter now with sickening incredulity.

'He's such a kind man,' I told Ian that evening. 'I feel so much better having seen him.'

As I spoke those words I brushed my fringe out of my eyes, and Ian noticed I had an angry red mark on the index finger of my right hand.

'Looks like Fiona's not the only one who's been in the wars,' he remarked. 'What happened there?'

'Oh, I'd forgotten about that. It happened on Tuesday night. One of the patients bit me.'

'What?' Ian said, horrified. 'I've known police colleagues of mine to get injured at work, but I didn't realise midwives got attacked, too. What on earth happened?'

I explained that I'd been in the middle of my night shift when I was sent down to Room Five, a first-stage room at the end of the corridor.

'Do you mind, Linda?' the sister had said. 'I know you'll be able to deal with her. Her name's Lisa Walters and she's in a bit of a state.'

I had a reputation for being calm and unflappable, even though very often I was feeling quite anxious inside. I obviously hid my feelings well as, according to my colleagues, I had a knack of transferring some of my cool composure to my patients.

I heard the young girl screaming before I went into the room, and was shocked by how distressed she looked as she writhed in agony on the bed.

'Help me!' she implored. 'Please help me. This is killin' me! Arrghhh! Arghhhh.'

I managed to get her to stop screaming long enough to tell me she had only started experiencing labour pains within the hour. Alarmingly, they had quickly accelerated from extremely mild period-like pains to the extremely intense labour she was now enduring.

'Let's have a look, shall we, Lisa?' I said gently. 'I'll just examine you and see how far you've got. I'm Linda, by the way …'

I took a step closer towards her and, to my surprise, the girl lurched at me and grabbed my hand. A split second later I felt her teeth sink into my finger.

'No, stop it!' I cried. 'Don't bite me!'

I actually pushed Lisa away from me and onto the bed because I was that startled. My finger was throbbing with the pain, and when I looked at it there were bite marks indented in my skin. Thankfully she hadn't drawn blood, but she'd come pretty close.

'I'm so sorry!' she blurted. 'I really am so AAAARRRRRRGGGGGGGHHHHHHHH! Help! I'm sorry! He-he-help me pleeeeeeese!'

'I will examine you now, but you must promise not to bite me again,' I scolded firmly. 'You really hurt me and I can't have any more of that behaviour.'

'Sorry, so sorry,' she repeated.

Lisa was already nine centimetres dilated. I took the decision to deliver her baby in this first-stage room, partly because her labour had progressed so rapidly and partly because I didn't trust how she would carry on should we have to transfer her to a delivery room.

It was a good decision, because literally within ten minutes she delivered a strapping little boy. He weighed just over nine pounds and Lisa had had no pain relief as there simply hadn't been time.

'Thank you, and I'm so sorry, Linda,' she said when she cradled her son in her arms. She looked very embarrassed as she said, 'Er, how's your hand?'

'You bit my finger, actually, but I'll live. I don't think I suffered as much pain as you, let's put it like that.'

'Will you have to tell anyone?'

'Yes, I'll have to put it in the notes, but that'll be the end of it. Don't you worry. You've got a lovely little boy. Perhaps if you have another baby you'll have to bring in a boiled sweet to bite on!'

Lisa smiled. 'Honestly, I've never bitten anyone or anything before. It was a moment of madness. The pain was so bad it made me go mental. Is that normal?'

'It can happen, and you had a particularly fast labour. Never mind. Put it out of your mind now and focus on your baby. What will you call him?'

'Gnasher,' she laughed slightly nervously. I think she was worried her little joke might offend me, but it didn't at all and I wished her the very best of luck with her baby, who she told me she would really be calling Spencer.

When Ian heard the story he couldn't believe how forgiving I was. 'You shouldn't have to put up with that in your place of work,' he said. 'Can't something be done about it?'

'Things like that happen,' I replied. 'We don't have rules and regulations about everything that can happen on a maternity ward; how can we? When a woman's in labour she can be so unpredictable. It's not such a big deal, is it?'

Ian looked unconvinced, but I just accepted it and moved on. If that happened today I'd react in exactly the same way – except now, of course, I would probably have to attend occupational health to be screened.

'Well, as long as you're all right, Linda,' Ian said.

'Oh I am,' I replied. 'I'm absolutely fine. Couldn't be happier, in fact.'

Chapter Ten

'I haven't felt the baby move'

In the mid-Eighties Ian and I bought a static caravan in Benllech Bay, Anglesey, and one summer we all learned to water-ski and loved it so much we saved up to buy a little speedboat. The children were really good at water-skiing, and we always had a ball whenever we went to the caravan site. Over the summer holidays I'd spend as much time as possible at the caravan, often just returning home to work my two evenings per week.

In term time the children did everything from Cubs and Brownies to swimming and dancing and Army Cadet training, and they often went to my parents' house for their tea after school. Of course, they had none of the electronic gadgets and computer games that children today have, but they'd make up their own games or play outside with balls and skipping ropes. Ian was often at work, but it didn't bother me. I liked nothing better than watching the children grow up happy.

'How's your day been?' he'd always ask me, to which I'd reply by telling him all about what the children got up to.

I didn't tell him much about my work, because even after being together for almost a decade by now, I always felt that I had to keep explaining my job to Ian because it was so very different to his. I found it a bit irritating, really, having to keep reminding him that in midwifery there are grey areas, and that feelings and intuition are more important than anything else.

I didn't even make an exception after a particularly memorable night at work, in October 1986. A lady called Nicola Bowman was admitted to the labour ward at thirty-eight weeks pregnant, and her story touched me very deeply. I knew Ian would find her story hard to understand, as it technically involved breaking hospital regulations, and so I didn't bother telling him. I think I told my mum instead, or maybe Sue Smith, as this was a story I felt I had to share.

'I haven't felt the baby move for two or three days,' Nicola said fearfully when she arrived on the ward. 'Do you think everything is all right?'

Nicola explained that she had booked an appointment at the antenatal clinic the following day, but had grown so concerned she'd asked her husband Nigel to drive her up the maternity unit at about 9 p.m., just as I started my shift.

'Let's have a little listen, shall we?' I said, settling her on a bed and running the Sonicaid foetal heart monitor over her abdomen. I knew it could be a source of great worry to a pregnant woman when her baby went quiet in the womb at this late stage in pregnancy, and such concerns were always taken very seriously. Thankfully, we nearly always found that the baby was fine and had probably decided to be active while the woman slept, when she was unaware of the movement.

Nigel stood hovering by the bedside, biting his nails. My heart went out to them both, it really did. This should be a time of great excitement and expectation, not dreadful worry. I didn't immediately pick up the baby's heartbeat and it was very quiet in the room. Nicola was holding her breath and I had to remind her to breathe normally as I continued moving the Sonicaid over her abdomen, seeking out the baby's heartbeat. I could feel Nigel's eyes trained on my hands and the monitor, no doubt desperately hoping it would beep into life any second now.

No sound or movement was forthcoming, and my own heart began to tighten. Nicola's worries were not unfounded; tragically her instincts had been correct. I checked and checked again, trying not to register my concern on my face, but there was silence. Nicola's baby had died in the womb and she would have to be told the dreadful news. 'Foetal death in utero' was the horrible, technical term that filled my head. I called the registrar, who came at once, and he checked my diagnosis.

'I am very, very sorry, but I cannot detect a heartbeat,' he told the couple. 'I'm afraid to tell you your baby has died in the womb. I'm so very sorry.'

The words clattered off the walls and hit Nicola and Nigel like missiles. They both gasped and held their hands over their mouths as the initial shock penetrated, and then they dissolved in each other's arms, trembling, crying and crumpling. Often on occasions like this, I think God helps a little. Nicola had to be induced. The process worked swiftly first time, her labour was quick and she coped incredibly well. Nobody spoke when the baby, a little boy, appeared. Nicola's cries of pain stopped as soon as the baby was delivered, and then there was nothing.

I knew from bitter experience that when a dead baby is delivered the silence is overwhelming and words seem meaningless. Nicola had Nigel to comfort her, and he was everything she needed right now. I gave her a nod and a half smile, to acknowledge that she had done well, but I didn't speak.

'Do you think we could have a little bit of time alone?' Nicola asked.

I had wrapped the little mite in a blanket and Nicola had indicated that she wanted to hold him. This was something midwives were taught to encourage by the Eighties, as research indicated that it helped women come to terms with the loss and helped with the grieving process.

I handed her the bundle. 'Of course,' I said. 'I'll be back in a little while.'

I left the room and walked across to the office. It was empty, thank goodness, and I stood by the sink and wept for several minutes. 'Right, Linda, come on now,' I told myself. 'Keep yourself together.'

I tapped quietly on the door and walked back into the labour room, having checked in the bathroom mirror that my cheeks were dry and my eyes were not too red or puffy. I wanted to put on a strong and brave face for Nicola; the last thing she needed was a tearful midwife to contend with.

To my surprise, Nicola was lying back on the bed and was alone in the room. There was no sign of Nigel or the baby.

'Wh-where's the ... where's your husband?' I asked tentatively.

'Don't be cross, Linda. We only live down the road from the hospital and I just wanted the baby to be in our house and in the room my husband and I had prepared, just one time.'

My eyes filled with tears again and I hugged Nicola closely. 'It's OK,' I said. 'It's OK.'

'He won't be long,' Nicola promised.

Nigel returned about twenty minutes later, holding the baby tightly to his chest, still wrapped in the hospital blanket. I had busied myself with writing up notes, offering words of comfort and trying to answer Nicola's many questions, but even so it seemed like an extremely long twenty minutes. I didn't ask Nigel any questions, and to this day I have no idea if he walked through the streets with the baby in his arms or drove him home in a car. Nigel told Nicola that everything was fine. Nobody had challenged him, and I was pleased the couple had got their wish. I would have to disclose this to the sister in charge, of course, but I was confident that there would be no repercussions, which indeed there weren't.

Nowadays midwives are obliged to ensure each baby has a suitable car seat in which to travel home, and each new mother is escorted out of the hospital with her child securely fastened in a carrier. Any man heading out of the unit with a baby in his arms would be confronted on safety grounds alone, and the chances of making it through the doors with a stillborn baby like that are absolutely zero.

This was a different era, however. The high-profile case of newborn Abbie Humphries, who was kidnapped from a maternity hospital in Nottingham by a woman posing as a nurse, would not hit the headlines until July 1994. That was almost eight years away, and at this time security at maternity units was simply not an issue. Visitors could walk in off the street and straight onto the wards without the need for a security pass or the press of a buzzer, and mothers thought nothing of leaving their baby unattended in a cot by the bed while they nipped to the toilet or even took a bath or shower. It was accepted that the other mothers on the ward would keep an eye on the baby and call a midwife if need be. The threat of anyone taking a baby from the maternity unit was simply unthinkable.

Hospital life was moving with the times in many other respects, however. In the late Eighties a new pay and grade system was brought into the NHS, which was known as the 'Agenda for Change'. It meant each worker was given a grade according to position and length of service. I was a Grade 6 staff nurse, which was not a low grade but meant my pay would be capped at a certain level. I was earning a good salary at that time and was not unhappy with my pay. In fact, I'd look at reports of rising unemployment on the television and consider myself very fortunate to have a secure job in the NHS, and it cushioned me from the recession.

When I saw things like the Toxteth riots taking place less than fifty miles away from me on the streets of Liverpool, with violent youths blaming Margaret Thatcher for robbing them of jobs and a future, it felt like a totally different world to the one I inhabited. Ian had more to do with the rioting, as some of his colleagues had to help the Merseyside Police, but I don't remember us talking much about it.

The NHS budget changes *did* have an impact on the running of the hospital, however. Gone were the golden days of the Seventies when disposable goods were plentiful and midwives used a thick sanitary towel to mop up a spillage because it was the nearest thing to hand and did the job effectively. Now everything from paper towels to bed linen was in much shorter supply, and the senior sister on the ward was accountable for every item ordered, a task she had to take very seriously.

Each department had a set budget for twelve months, and midwives were constantly reminded of this fact. 'Don't leave piles of nappies on display, because if the women see plentiful supplies they will help themselves to a handful,' the night sister would remind us.

Disposable nappies had almost completely replaced the old fashioned terry nappies in the hospital by this time, although some women still preferred the cloth nappies as they were cheaper than disposables. I occasionally saw hospital nappies blowing on washing lines around the area. You couldn't miss them as they had a big green stripe down the side and the words 'Tameside Hospital Property' printed on them. We knew that if women were prepared to take terry nappies they would certainly not pass up the chance of some free disposables, if they could readily help themselves.

Baby milk was still given out free, though that was a luxury that would eventually dry up in subsequent budget cuts, and by 2009 mothers had to supply their own formula milk if they were not breastfeeding, as we only kept emergency supplies on the ward from then on. Of course, we were strongly recommending breastfeeding as part of our 'breast is best' campaign by that time, too, which was another reason not to give out free formula milk.

One exception to the frugal rule was with disposable plastic gloves, which were always in plentiful supply in the Eighties. AIDS had first been identified in 1981, but it wasn't until 1986 that the majority of Britons became fully aware of it through an exceptionally high-profile and hard-hitting publicity campaign. Millions of leaflets were delivered to households up and down the country, and a memorable television advert told viewers: 'Don't die of ignorance' and showed a tombstone with the letters AIDS engraved on it.

I was not alone in being alarmed by the Government's publicity drive and, even though it was not the intention to scare people, there was a lot of uncertainty and fear generated by the powerful coverage. Many people were afraid that AIDS could be transmitted in the workplace, and there was quite a bit of panic that infected patients could easily transmit the disease to doctors and nurses, and vice versa. The result was that it was drummed into midwives like me to wear disposable gloves at every opportunity.

'Even if the baby has to pop out first, don't touch it until you've got your gloves on,' I remember one of my superiors cautioning.

The campaign was so alarming that nurses and midwives became frightened of handling needles, worrying about 'needle stick injuries' as we call them, which might infect us. Some reporting was very misleading, as it had people believing that just breathing the same air or shaking someone's hand could transmit AIDS, which we soon learned was utter nonsense. Nevertheless, I did as I was told, and disposable gloves became a vital part of the midwife's standard kit.

The whole issue of HIV/AIDS changed the way we practised, in fact, which I sometimes did not think was a good thing. However, rules are rules and this is just one of the many changes I have had to accept as society has changed over the years. I also understand, of course, that the pregnant women themselves may prefer to have this barrier between themselves and medical professionals, which I respect.

A more positive change, in my view, was in how pregnant teenagers were treated. When I first started out in midwifery there was a great deal of shame attached to teenage pregnancy. Back in the Sixties and Seventies it was much less common to encounter such pregnancies, and I can remember how awkward and embarrassing it used to be when a teenager came into the antenatal clinic. You could almost feel the shame following them into the room, and often girls were so terrified they didn't tell their parents until very late in the pregnancy, which meant they did not have any antenatal care.

Now, though, girls were much less embarrassed about it, and their parents seemed to be generally more tolerant, too, with more mothers loyally holding their daughters' hands at clinics and in the delivery rooms. As far as I could see the shift was partly due to the fact couples were starting to live together more before marriage, and so we were beginning to see more unmarried mothers of all ages. This seemed to lessen the stigma for the pregnant teenagers, although of course prejudice still existed, just as it does today.

For this reason, I always made an extra special effort to treat pregnant teenagers with respect and courtesy. It would have been awful if a young girl felt she was being judged by her midwife, and I tried to make each one feel special, just as I believe every pregnant woman should.

In the spring of 1989 I arrived at work one night to be told there was a teenager labouring in the first-stage room, who would be my first patient of the evening.

I entered the room and found a young woman called Tricia Drake lying quietly on the bed. A quick look at her notes had told me she was eighteen years old, and to my surprise she had a wedding band on her finger, next to a pretty little solitaire engagement ring.

'Will I be long? My hubby's on his way,' she said. 'Sorry, where are my manners? I'm Tricia. Pleased to meet you.'

'I'm pleased to meet you, too. I'm Linda. Let's have a look, shall we? So, your waters went a few hours ago and you're having contractions about five minutes apart?'

'Yes, that's right. It's hurting, but I think I'm doing OK.'

As I carried out the examination I gave myself a little ticking off. I had expected such a young girl to be unmarried, and I had also imagined she might be accompanied by her mother, as was typically the case with a teenager. As it turned out Tricia had been brought into the hospital by her father, who had now gone to fetch his son-in-law from work, as he didn't have a car and normally got a lift home with a mate after his night shift at a distribution centre in Ashton.

'Kenny's so excited!' Tricia told me. 'It's probably just as well he's not driving himself. When I phoned his work before he was absolutely buzzing!'

I was so pleased that Tricia was not the archetypal single mum I'd imagined she might be, who'd got herself pregnant by mistake or perhaps wouldn't have a partner to support her. You'd have thought I'd have known after all these years that you can never predict *anything* in the maternity unit, and I smiled to myself as I realised this was one of those pleasant surprises. If I hadn't seen her date of birth I might not have guessed she was a teenager at all, in fact, as Tricia seemed so mature and poised.

'I don't think Kenny will miss a thing,' I reassured Tricia. 'I think you might have a long night ahead.'

'Oh, that's good,' she replied. 'Thanks, Linda.'

'Most women groan when I say they have a long night ahead,' I smiled.

'Well, you know what I mean. I want Kenny here with me. My mum wanted to come, too, but I've put her off. She says she has such fond memories of the hospital, would you believe!'

'Does she now! That's something I don't hear often, either!'

'Well, she gave birth to me and my brother and sister in here, and I suppose it was a bit special … oh, brilliant! Here he is!'

Kenny appeared at the door, breathless and wide-eyed with excitement.

'Legged it across the car park,' he panted. 'Can I come in? How's it going?'

'Of course you can come in,' I replied. 'In fact, you can sit with your wife and time her contractions for me if you like. She's doing very well, and for the time being she just needs your company and support. I'll be back to check on you soon, Tricia.'

I left the young couple alone for a while and attended to two other admissions before deciding it was time to move Tricia into the delivery room. She had progressed really well, to seven centimetres dilatation, and had done so relatively easily, as is often the case with such a young woman.

It warmed my heart to see how attentive and caring Kenny was. He wiped Tricia's brow with a damp flannel and had even taken the trouble to put together a cassette tape of her favourite music, which he'd packed in her hospital bag as a surprise, complete with a little Phillips tape machine. He politely asked my permission before playing the tape, which he'd compiled by recording a pop show on the radio. The first song he played was 'Especially for You' by Kylie Minogue and Jason Donovan, which ended very suddenly when Madonna's 'Like a Prayer' came crashing in. 'Sorry, fingers weren't fast enough!' Kenny smirked, explaining how he'd recorded the tunes while he was painting the walls in the baby's nursery, and had to keep running up and down the ladder to press 'pause' on the cassette recorder each time the DJ spoke between tracks. Spots of white paint on the tape machine were testament to his tale.

Tricia thought this was hysterically funny, no doubt partly because she was sucking hard on gas and air by this point. As 'Like a Prayer' was cut off unceremoniously, making way for the second chorus of 'Eternal Flame' by the Bangles, Tricia now had the urge to push.

'What do you want me to do?' Kenny panicked.

'Just hold my hand. Huuuuuurrrrggghhhh!'

'That's it,' I soothed. 'When I tell you, give a nice big push Tricia. You're doing ever so well. Ever so well. Yes, there we are …'

Just six minutes later a bonny little girl emerged into my waiting hands.

'What is it?' Kenny asked as the warm bundle I lifted aloft cried loudly.

'A baby!' Tricia puffed.

'A baby girl!' I said. 'Congratulations!'

'Well done!' Kenny beamed. 'Wow! Well done!' He looked shell-shocked but absolutely smitten as he watched me swiftly clean up the little girl and hand her to her mum for a cuddle.

Tricia's face was a picture. She had tears rolling down her cheeks as she introduced herself to her daughter. 'I'm your mummy,' she said. 'Yes I am. I'm your mummy.'

The little girl weighed a healthy seven pounds, nine ounces and was so fair she looked bald. She had stopped crying within moments of being in her mother's arms.

'You are beautiful,' Tricia told her. She stroked each of her daughter's tiny wriggling fingers and kissed her downy head several times. 'Look at your eyelashes!' she told the little girl. 'Aren't you the lucky one?' I peeped over and saw that the baby had long, white-blonde eyelashes. She really was a delightful little thing. I had a lump in my throat, but little did I know that the high emotions of this birth were not over yet.

'Shall I go and phone your mum?' Kenny suggested eventually.

'Yes, please,' Tricia said. 'She'll be dying to hear. Tell her not to worry, it wasn't triplets!'

'She didn't think you had more than one in there, did she?' I asked jokily.

'No! But I was glad to have my first scan to make sure. But with me being a triplet it was the first thing everyone talked about when I found out I was pregnant.'

'You're a triplet? Oh, I didn't realise ...'

Kenny reappeared, interrupting me.

'Spoke to your mum, and your dad. She's thrilled to bits, they both are,' he told Tricia. 'Or, to use your dad's words, they're as "chuffed as mint balls". He's driving her in as soon as visiting starts in the morning.'

Kenny stepped up to his daughter and said softly: 'Watch out little one, grandma Geraldine and granddad Mick are coming to see you! But you don't need to worry, they'll be the proudest grandparents in all of Ashton-under-Lyne.'

A light went on in my head. It lit up a shadowy corner of my brain, where I saw a man called Mick use that very phrase – 'chuffed as mint balls' – many years earlier. I saw Mick Drew and his wife Geraldine, who had just given birth naturally to triplets, in the old maternity unit at Ashton General. It must have been 1971, because I remember thinking it was a shame that Geraldine missed out on giving birth in here, as the new unit wasn't quite ready to open.

One of the babies, the first-born daughter, I had delivered myself, and she was so fair she looked as bald as an egg. She looked precisely like Tricia's newborn baby girl, in fact.

I gasped and was unable to stop a tear rolling down my cheek as my memories crystallised. 'Are you all right?' Kenny asked.

'Yes, yes I am,' I said as I tried to compose myself, and asked him softly if his mother-in-law was called Geraldine Drew. 'Yes, she is. She's great. Her and Mick are the salt of the earth, best in-laws you could wish for. Do you know them, then?'

'Yes, I believe I do,' I replied. 'Let's just get Tricia and the baby settled on the postnatal ward and I will come up and see you later. By the way, do you happen to know if Tricia was the first triplet to be born?'

'Yes I was!' she called over, without looking up. 'How did you know?'

'I'll tell you later.'

I had to sit down for several minutes in the kitchen to gather my thoughts. I had just delivered the child of a woman I had also delivered, eighteen years earlier! What were the chances? It was absolutely incredible. I could picture myself clearly, my youthful face shining, as I stepped up and delivered baby Tricia in a packed delivery suite in the old maternity unit at Ashton General. Geraldine was magnificent, giving birth to her three healthy babies naturally. There was Tricia, then a brother, and then another girl, with more hair than her sister. The birth of the triplets caused quite a sensation at the time. I had never forgotten it, though I'd not seen hide nor hair of the family in all these years.

At the end of my shift I slipped into the postnatal ward, where I found Tricia taking a nap. Kenny was sitting in the chair beside her bed, watching over their daughter as she also slept.

'I can't *tell* you how delighted I am to have delivered your daughter,' I told Kenny.

'We're both very grateful,' he said. 'It couldn't have gone better, Linda. Thank you so much.'

I steeled myself and told Kenny that I had worked something out that was just a little bit special.

'You might find this hard to believe ... but I delivered Tricia,' I told him. 'I was one of the team who delivered the triplets, and I delivered Tricia. I remember it very clearly.'

Kenny's jaw dropped open, and at that moment Tricia began to stir.

'Did I hear that right, or am I dreaming?' she said, propping herself up.

'No, honestly. It's true. Your brother was born second and was breech, and your sister was the last one born. I also remember you have three older siblings. How is the family?'

Between them Tricia and Kenny told me that Mick and Geraldine were both as 'right as rain', recently having celebrated their twenty-fifth wedding anniversary with a stay in a posh hotel in Scotland, paid for by all six children. The other two triplets still lived at home, and it sounded like Kenny had been welcomed into the family so much he was practically treated like a seventh sibling.

'Lots of people said Kenny and I were too young to get married,' Tricia confided. 'But my mum and dad met when they were only sixteen. They both told us: "If you love each other, that's what matters most." They've been great. They'll be so thrilled to hear this!'

I asked Tricia to give her parents my regards. I was not on duty again until the following week, when Tricia had been discharged, and I never saw any of the family again, but knowing they were all happy and healthy was what mattered most.

'Do you know what, Linda?' one of my colleagues joked when I told her the tale. 'If you keep working here you might get to deliver a *third* generation of Drews.'

I laughed, thinking that really was beyond the realms of possibility.

'I expect I'll be long retired by then,' I told my colleague, but of course, it's now twenty-three years since Tricia and Kenny had their daughter, and here I am, still practising.

Chapter Eleven

'I was hoping to apply for a community post'

At the end of 1989 I was still working two nights a week on the postnatal ward, and I was enjoying it more than ever. Jonathan and Fiona were both in secondary school by this time and it was much easier for me to sleep during the day, now they were older and didn't need collecting at the school gate.

Unfortunately, despite the fact that my life as a parent was becoming easier, my personal life had become more problematic, because my relationship with Ian was not in good shape. Rather like with Graham, it's very difficult to pinpoint exactly when and how things started to go wrong. There wasn't a dramatic event that changed things for Ian and me. It was far more subtle than that. Looking back, I think throughout the latter part of the Eighties, as each year went by, I started to become more aware of how little we had in common.

As I wrote the previous few chapters of this book, I realised I have very few memories of Ian and me really being together as a married couple in the late Eighties. We didn't share very many hobbies or interests, we had some quite separate groups of friends and we didn't even like watching the same programmes on television. Our personalities were so very different, and perhaps as we became older our distinct traits became more noticeable.

I'd turned forty in 1988 and was at that age when I really knew who I was and what I wanted. I liked it when life was rolling gently by with everybody getting along, having a few laughs along the way and feeling content and comfortable together. Stability and peace have always been important to me.

As the children grew up, however, it had become apparent that Ian had quite different ideas, especially when it came to parenting. As you might expect from a policeman, Ian was much stricter than me, and there seemed to be a lot of tension and conflict in the house. I wasn't happy, and I don't think Ian could have been, either.

My job, as always, provided a constant source of stimulation and satisfaction, and as my personal life faltered I began to think about working more hours. I enjoyed nights, but after more than a decade on night duty, and with the children becoming rapidly more independent, I considered applying to do longer hours, on day duty. My ultimate dream was to work out in the district, as a community midwife as I had done in my training with Mrs Tattersall, but I knew you could only do that if you worked at least four days a week.

My only concern about applying for day duty was that it might mean working permanently on the postnatal ward, which mostly involved teaching new mums to breastfeed and bathe their babies, and making sure the mums and babies were fit and well enough to be discharged. I knew I would miss delivering babies, and I wondered if the postnatal ward might be less of a joy than I was used to, having been on the labour ward for so many years. I decided not to rush into anything, as I really wasn't sure what to do.

'Let me tell you, Nurse, I've never been so embarrassed in my whole life!' a patient called Michelle told me one night, after I had popped up to the postnatal ward to see another lady I'd delivered earlier, on my night shift.

Michelle was a very large lady, weighing at least twenty stone. Her baby, Samantha, was a little six-pounder who looked like a doll in her mother's vast arms.

'Honest to God, I can laugh about it now but at the time it were no joke.'

'What happened?' I asked gamely. I'd already heard on the grapevine what had gone on, but it was clear Michelle wanted to tell me the story from start to finish, and so I sat on the chair at the side of her bed and listened.

'Well, when I got here I was practically ready to push, but I were bursting for a wee. I said to the midwife, I said: "I've got to go," and she helped me onto the toilet. Well, it were as funny as anything. As soon as I parked me backside on the bog I just had to push. The midwife was telling me to hurry up and get off the loo, but I just couldn't get up. She had to call for back-up, she did! It took two of 'em to lift me off in the end, and they only just managed it in time. Any longer and poor little Sammy would have landed in the toilet. Can you imagine! Honest to God, it were touch and go!'

I enjoyed the story very much and couldn't help being reminded of some of the near misses I'd been involved in when patients of mine had taken themselves to the toilet during labour. The baby who was born in a bowl on the floor of the toilet, when I was a rather over-confident new midwife, was going through my head, but I didn't say a word about it to Michelle, as I didn't want to take anything away from her funny tale.

Michelle thought her birth story was the most dramatic and hilarious one ever, and that was exactly how it should be.

In fact, I thought that with women like her, perhaps I might have the best of both worlds if I did work permanently on the postnatal ward. I wouldn't have hands-on experience of delivering babies, but nor would I have the intense pressure I sometimes felt on the labour ward. I could enjoy the babies and the birth stories, without so much stress for a while. Maybe it was just what I needed, what with my marriage difficulties at home.

Ian and I eventually split up at the start of 1991, and I don't think I fully realised how much our relationship had deteriorated until I was living as a single woman. I actually felt so free it was like I was on holiday every day. I remember saying as much to the postman one morning, and he pulled my leg. 'Can you see seagulls and the sand, Mrs Fairley?' he teased cheekily.

I don't wish to be critical of Ian. It was a mutual decision to split up, and I would like to think that he felt equally liberated by our separation. I don't blame him for things not working out between us, either. We were simply two very different people, and the longer we spent together the more those differences became apparent.

Paying a mortgage on my own was not going to be feasible with me still working just two nights a week, and as soon as Ian and I had agreed to go our separate ways and file for divorce it gave me the push I needed to finally ask to come off night duty and increase my hours.

I asked to see Miss Travis, who was now head of midwifery. She had taken over from Miss O'Neil, who in turn had succeeded Miss Sefton in this role. As I tapped on Miss Travis's door and asked her secretary if it would be possible to make an appointment, I was transported right back to the day of my interview to become a pupil midwife in 1969. It seemed unbelievable to me that more than two decades had passed since that life-changing day.

Miss Sefton and her then-deputy, Miss O'Neil, appeared like characters from another era in my mind. They were both old-school, no-nonsense, matronly figures. It hardly seemed possible that here I was, all these years on, still doing the same job while now working under my third head of midwifery!

I didn't think I'd changed one bit, but of course I had. Back then I was a meek and inexperienced young woman, recently married and with long chestnut hair that shone as brightly as my new wedding ring. Now I was a self-assured, experienced forty-three-year-old, recently separated, and with more than a couple of grey hairs in my head.

One thing that had not changed in all those years was my love of midwifery. It's what brought me here in December 1969, and it's what brought me to this door again, in March 1991. I still loved my job as passionately as I did as a pupil midwife; the only difference was that now I needed it, more than ever.

Miss Travis seemed extremely approachable, but that didn't stop me feeling a little anxious. After all, I had a big question to ask, and paying the mortgage depended on it.

'Miss Travis will see you right away,' the secretary said, which took me by surprise. I'd expected to be told to wait, or to be given an appointment to return to later.

I entered the office and Miss Travis greeted me with a very welcoming smile. As the maternity unit is not big, most of the staff usually know a fair bit about each other's business, and it soon became apparent that Miss Travis had guessed why I wanted to see her.

'I was wondering if I might be able to increase my hours, only …'

'Yes of course, Linda. I understand. What do you want to do and when do you want to start?'

I was astonished it was that simple, and in the spur of the moment I took the opportunity to ask for more than I'd intended to.

'Four days please,' I replied, unable to suppress a grin. 'And I was hoping to apply for a community post, when one comes available.'

'I can put you up to four days on the postnatal ward immediately, and I shall take note of your interest in the community. How does that sound?'

'Ideal. Thank you very much indeed!'

I couldn't believe it. A community post had appealed to me for a long time, although I'd never asked about the possibility before as I knew very well that community midwives had to do a four-day week, which hadn't suited me until now. I would not have asked for it today had Miss Travis not been so accommodating, and now I was thrilled to bits.

I'd never forgotten my exciting first forays into the district with Mrs Tattersall as a pupil midwife, riding my moped across cobbled streets to addresses scattered all over Ashton. There was something very down to earth yet at the same time incredibly exciting about this type of midwifery. It was so very different to delivering a baby in the clinical, sterile surroundings of the hospital. You never quite knew what you would find in each woman's home. Who would be there with her? Where would she be labouring? And of course, the biggest question of all: How many cups of tea would the father-to-be brew? That was something Mrs Tattersall and I laughed about so many times, because every expectant dad seemed to launch himself into tea-making mode the minute his wife went into labour, and very often didn't stop nipping out to put the kettle on until after the baby was born.

I didn't have to wait long for a post to become available. I was interviewed in September 1991 and was offered to start work as a community midwife in the November. It felt like the pieces of my life were falling back into place quickly after my marriage breakdown.

Coming off nights in the meantime actually proved to be very enjoyable, too. I did several months on the postnatal ward as I waited for my community post to begin and, as I'd hoped, I did appreciate spending time with the new mums without experiencing the high drama of the labour ward. I missed delivering babies, but I made the most of the calmness for a few months, knowing I would soon be out in the district.

My increased hours meant I could comfortably afford a mortgage of my own, and I moved into a three-bedroom house in Meadway, Stalybridge, with Jonathan and Fiona. Stuart had already moved into his own place by this point, and was working at a travel agency in Romiley. Everybody seemed settled, and I felt very happy about the changes in my life.

As November approached I was *very* excited about the prospect of working in the community again. It felt so right for me, and I just knew I would love it. Building a relationship with the expectant mum, sharing her journey and being a part of the miracle of birth was what I enjoyed most of all about being a midwife. Yes, I adored giving the babies a cuddle and a bath, or helping the new mums establish breastfeeding on the postnatal ward. It was a very rewarding part of the job, but in the long term I wanted more. I wanted to get to know the mums in the exciting build-up to the birth. I wanted to be there with them when labour started, and more than anything I longed to feel the warmth of a newborn emerging into my hands once more.

I will never forget my very first day out in the district, because I was reminded straightaway of the very warm welcome the community midwife typically receives. When I was a pupil midwife, shadowing Mrs Tattersall on her rounds, I'd enjoyed seeing the smile spread across people's faces when they announced appreciatively: 'The midwife's here!' It made me feel very proud of my job, and it made me realise how important the role of the community midwife is.

Now it was early in the morning of 25 November and I was listening to GMR, a local BBC radio station, on my car stereo as I approached Shirebrook Park in Glossop. Although Glossop is technically in Derbyshire, it fell within the radius of my rounds, and still does today. I'd been called out to a lady who was having her third baby at home, and the house was up in the hills.

I remember hearing the engine of the little red Fiesta I drove at that time straining up the country roads, and I felt a little anxious that I might break down. It was just coming up to 6 a.m. and was very dark and cold, and there were very few cars on the road. In those days I had no mobile telephone. Mobiles were just about in use by then, but were very expensive and were about the size of a house brick, and nobody I knew had one.

I had no SatNav either, as that was many years away from being invented. This meant it was just me and my little A–Z street map, out there in the wintry morning air, driving to the aid of a pregnant woman. I didn't feel so very different to how

I'd felt as a student, riding my moped through the streets of Ashton in 1970 to meet Mrs Tattersall at the home of a labouring mother. I still had the same adrenaline running through my body, filling me with a mixture of excitement and nervous anticipation about how the delivery would go, or whether I would actually get there in one piece, or indeed in time for the birth. I was in my element then, and I was now. One difference was that I was on my own now, but that didn't alarm me. I had two decades of experience under my belt to help me cope with whatever the day would bring, and though Mrs Tattersall was not with me in person, I never forgot her words of wisdom.

When the 6 a.m. news came on my car radio I was dismayed to hear that Freddie Mercury, lead singer of Queen, had died of AIDS the night before. I wasn't a Queen fan, but I'd loved some of their greatest hits like 'Bohemian Rhapsody' and 'Don't Stop Me Now'. I think the news distracted me somewhat, because it wasn't until I eventually arrived at the address and parked up outside the house several minutes later that I realised one of my tyres was flat. The car hadn't felt quite right but I'd put it down to the hilly climb. It wasn't until I felt the car wobble and buckle a little beneath me as I pulled into the kerb that I realised what was wrong.

Lifting a delivery pack out of the boot, I silently acknowledged that I would have to sort that problem out later: Mrs Leadbetter's third baby was the priority right now; there was no time to think about the flat tyre. As I approached the large detached house I noticed the curtains twitching in the bedroom window of the house next door. The neighbour, a middle-aged man, gave me a smile and a nod when I caught his eye.

Mrs Leadbetter was forty-one years old and married to a bank manager. It had been made clear to her that, being over forty, she was not an ideal candidate for a home birth, as older women were considered to have a higher risk of developing complications and she might indeed end up delivering in hospital. According to her notes, Mrs Leadbetter had put it in writing that she would take responsibility if the birth did not go to plan, and as a result her home birth had been agreed by one of my superiors. Unfortunately, Mrs Leadbetter had then gone three weeks overdue and had refused to be induced, meaning we now had two indications running against us – her age as well as her being extremely overdue. What with the bitter cold and the sad news on the radio, not to mention my flat tyre, I found myself shivering and feeling a little frazzled when I rang the bell.

I felt instantly better when Mr Leadbetter answered the door, however. He greeted me like a long-lost relative, and though he did not actually sing out: 'the midwife's here!' as I'd heard so many others do in the past, he might just as well have done.

'Do come in!' he said enthusiastically. 'I am *so* glad to see you!' He shook my hand firmly, offered to carry my bag and showed me briskly up the stairs to the master bedroom of his smart, spacious home. I couldn't help smiling. This was what I loved about this job. I was back in the community and in the heart of this home on such a special day. It was a huge privilege.

'Belinda is being very brave indeed. Here she is!'

Mr Leadbetter pushed open the bedroom door, placed my bag inside and said: 'I'll leave you ladies to it. Tea, anybody?'

I was pleased to see that Mrs Leadbetter appeared to be doing very well indeed. She managed to give me a smile and thank me for coming, even though she was panting quite a bit. I noticed her breaths came in a very controlled way, which somehow seemed to fit in with the whole environment I'd walked into. The bedroom was absolutely immaculate with not a speck of dust in sight, or an item out of place.

Beside the bed there was a copy of Dr Benjamin Spock's *Baby and Child Care*, which had a bookmark neatly tucked in the back cover, almost as if Mrs Leadbetter had reached the final page just in time to give birth. Clearly, she was an extremely organised lady. Her bed linen appeared freshly laundered and pressed, and the thick cream carpet beneath my feet still had tracks in it where the Hoover had been pushed around.

'I hope this is not a false alarm, but I think things are happening,' Mrs Leadbetter told me, looking extremely pleased with herself. 'I think I am almost about to push! Poof poof pooooooofffff! I'd like to have this baby out before Thomas and William wake up for nursery and school. Foooof. Ooof. Ooooooooof.'

I smiled as I prepared to examine Mrs Leadbetter, thinking she may be being a little ambitious to think she could deliver this baby precisely at her convenience. I noted that she'd placed several large towels and a plastic sheet beneath her, to protect the luxurious bedding, and I sincerely hoped all her best-laid plans would come to fruition as she wished.

'Let's have a look, shall we? Goodness! I can see the head. Well done, Mrs Leadbetter. You're right. It *is* time to push. Just keep breathing steadily for a moment whilst I get my delivery pack opened. You're doing really, really well.'

Mr Leadbetter arrived with two glasses of fruit juice, and apologised for not making a cup of tea. 'I think we're out of tea leaves,' he explained, which prompted Mrs Leadbetter to gasp in alarm as well as pain as a long contraction gripped her abdomen.

'I – need – to – push,' Mrs Leadbetter intoned politely, biting her lips bravely.

Mr Leadbetter hovered at the side of the bed, wringing his hands and tapping one of his feet, which was clad in a dark brown suede slipper. He stayed like that for several minutes, peering in amazement at his wife as she gave just four extremely controlled pushes before a warm, noisy little boy emerged into my hands. Being overdue, the baby's skin was a little dry and wrinkled, as the protective vernix covering his body had been absorbed during his extra time in the womb. His fingernails and toenails were longer than usual, but he was a sturdy and handsome little chap with a mop of thick black hair.

'Congratulations, Mrs Leadbetter! You did ever so well. It's a boy!'

I went to wrap the baby in a towel but Mrs Leadbetter indicated that she wanted him placed directly on her chest. 'Read an article,' she smiled, gazing adoringly at her son as she held out her arms to take hold of him. 'Skin-to-skin is good for bonding.'

This was something midwives were becoming increasingly aware of at this time. The many benefits of skin-to-skin care were several years away from being fully acknowledged in the UK, but so-called 'Kangaroo Care' was nothing new. A Colombian paediatrician called Edgar Rey had first used the term in 1978, when inadequate incubator care in the hospital where he worked prompted him to encourage women to effectively 'incubate' their own babies by snuggling them to their bare chests. This proved effective for maintaining the baby's body temperature as well as encouraging bonding and breastfeeding.

Mrs Leadbetter was clearly an educated woman who had read up on the subject, and I was very pleased she had. Her newborn son's initial noisy cries subsided into a contented snuffle as he nestled into his mother's chest. As if by magic, he latched on and began to breastfeed immediately. There was no fuss or anxiety and none of the awkwardness that often accompanied a baby's first attempts at breastfeeding. It was a wonderful, heart-warming sight, and I couldn't help thinking what a far cry this was from the days when Mrs Tattersall placed the baby in the cot a few minutes after the birth, and then thought nothing of sharing a cigarette with a new mother.

Mr Leadbetter kissed his wife tenderly on the forehead as she continued to breastfeed. 'Well done, darling,' he said before kissing the baby, too.

'What will you call him?' I asked.

'Possibly Peter,' they replied in unison, before bursting into peals of laughter.

Mr Leadbetter explained that they had talked at length about choosing the name Peter should they have a third little boy, but their response showed they were still both a little undecided. About half an hour after she gave birth, Mrs Leadbetter felt able to get up and go to the bathroom, and she placed 'possibly Peter' in a beautiful mahogany swinging crib beside her bed.

'Will you help me change the sheets quickly?' I asked Mr Leadbetter. 'We can have it done before your wife gets back.'

He looked a little surprised, but dutifully helped me remove the bloodied towels and replace the fitted sheet. He then took the soiled laundry downstairs, and was out of the room when Mrs Leadbetter returned.

'Oh, thank you!' she said as she settled back into the freshly made bed. 'You did that very quickly.'

'Your husband helped,' I replied, which prompted yet more peals of laughter from Mrs Leadbetter. 'How did you manage to get him to do that?' she snorted. 'I'm absolutely flabbergasted.'

It turned out that Mr Leadbetter never lifted a finger around the home. He had never once made the bed before, and Mrs Leadbetter said she wouldn't mind betting that the reason we'd only had orange juice instead of tea earlier had nothing to do with the fact there were no tea leaves in the house; Mr Leadbetter probably couldn't find them, as he rarely put the kettle on either.

'How on earth did you get him to help?' she asked.

'I just asked, and I suppose he didn't like to say no,' I giggled. 'Men don't tend to argue with midwives!'

We were both laughing our heads off when he reappeared a few minutes later with the two little brothers in tow, who stared in wonderment at the sleeping little bundle of joy that had arrived whilst they slept. 'What time is your mother arriving?' Mr Leadbetter asked his wife rather forlornly.

'Don't panic, any minute now,' Mrs Leadbetter replied, looking at her bedside clock. It was almost 9 a.m. and, as everything was as it should be, I would be on my way shortly. I didn't need Mrs Leadbetter to explain that her husband was relying on his mother-in-law to keep the house ticking over while she recovered from the birth; that was obvious. Mr

Leadbetter was clearly one of those high-achieving and no doubt high-earning males who held down a fantastic job and, in return, was absolved of any responsibility in the home.

As I said goodbye to 'possibly Peter' and his family and walked down the garden path, I suddenly remembered about my puncture. It had completely slipped my mind, and my first thought was that if Mr Leadbetter couldn't even make a cup of tea he was unlikely to be able to help me change a tyre. I was just wondering what I was going to do next when Mr Leadbetter darted out of the house in his fancy slippers and caught me up on the path.

'Totally forgot,' he blustered. 'Donald next door changed your tyre. Colin opposite helped. They saw you arrive. Lucky you had a spare. Hope you don't mind, you left your key in the hall and when Donald knocked it wasn't a good time to interrupt ...'

'That's so kind,' I beamed. 'Is Donald the man next door, at number 46? I saw him looking out the window when I pulled up.'

I drove away on a real high that morning. What an uplifting experience 'possibly Peter's' birth had been, and what wonderful neighbours the Leadbetters had. Donald and Colin had both gone off to work, but I would call and thank them personally when I came back for one of my home visits. They had really put the icing on the cake for me that day, and I felt terrific. I had found my niche, I was sure of it. It was like my whole life had been leading up to this point, and this was what I was destined to do.

Chapter Twelve

'Shoo you great oaf!'

Out in the district, I was very fortunate to work in a team with two other community midwives called Betty Simpson and Carol Porteus. Betty was ten years older than me and had a very motherly disposition and a matronly figure to match. She had short grey hair, a smiley face and a bad knee that meant she couldn't kneel down very easily. Betty had four grown-up children and had entered midwifery later in life, but she was a complete natural in the job. Carol, on the other hand, was ten years younger than me and was slim and pretty with it. She was extremely modern in her outlook, articulate and forth-right, too. Married to a Ghanaian called Asam, she had two young children and lived in Stockport.

Between us I reckon we made a great team. Betty was a solid, dependable force who was a realist and always kept our feet on the ground, while Carol was very forward-thinking and constantly had her eye on how we could improve our service and change with the times. I felt very comfortable working with both of them. I was forty-three years old by now and was probably something of a mixture between the two of them, having been a midwife for more than twenty years but still being young enough to feel constantly excited and chal-lenged by my job, particularly as I was re-learning the ropes out in the community after so many years in the maternity unit.

'I'm really glad I'm working with you,' Carol said during my first week as a community midwife. I'll never forget it. I was in the kitchen near the labour ward and Carol had appeared with a copy of the rota, which we call the 'off duty', in her hand.

'That's a nice thing to say,' I smiled. I was just about to go on and thank her for giving me such a warm welcome when she added, 'I know your children are older and your uterus is in the bin.'

So much for the compliment, but Carol went on to explain that, as her children were still very young, she would like to have the school holidays off and was glad that I was past that stage with my family and would not be competing with her to work term-time only. This was true, as Jonathan was seventeen and Fiona thirteen by now.

'I see what you mean,' I grinned, warming instantly to my new straight-talking colleague. To this day, Carol says she can't remember uttering that phrase to me, but she honestly did and I still rib her about it occasionally. She is now a very successful senior tutor on the Midwifery degree course at Manchester University, and I joke that I'm pleased the demise of my own childbearing years might have played some small part in helping Carol on her way!

Between us Betty, Carol and I planned the off-duty so that we each had one day off one week then three the next, including the weekend, with two of us working on any given day. When Carol and I were on duty together we would speak at 8.30 p.m. in the evenings when her children were in bed, dividing up the jobs and deciding who was visiting which patient. When I was paired with Betty we spoke in the morning at 8.30 a.m., as neither of us had children to take to school and it suited us both better.

The diary was always full, as at that time we were required to visit each new mother every day for ten days after the birth. There were also eight GP practices across Glossop where between us we ran a weekly antenatal clinic at every surgery. Each of us carried a pager, which we called a 'bleep', so that if the maternity unit needed to divert us to an imminent delivery we could always be contacted.

Hearing my bleep go off never failed to raise my heart rate, as I never knew how urgent the call would be. A contact number would flash up and I would need to get to a telephone as soon as possible. Needless to say, an urgent call always superseded a routine home visit.

I remember receiving such a call whilst visiting Mrs Leadbetter when 'possibly Peter' was three days old. Unexpectedly, Mrs Leadbetter was in tears when I arrived. It's certainly not uncommon for a woman to become tearful in the days after giving birth because her hormones are all over the place, and of course she is coming to terms with the reality of her huge responsibility just when she is feeling physically weak. Day three is well known for being the most unstable time for a new mother, as the hormone balance is at its most precarious.

'It's what we call the baby blues,' I was saying to Mrs Leadbetter when my bleep went off. 'It's perfectly normal. Do you not remember feeling the same way with Thomas, or William?'

'No! I don't. Everything was perfect with those two. I feel so silly, but I can't help it!'

'Honestly, don't worry. Every birth is different. I was quite blue with my first baby, and then everything was fine with my daughter. It didn't last long at all.'

Mrs Leadbetter wiped her wet eyes, smearing her neatly applied mascara down her cheeks.

'I'm sure you're right. At least "possibly Peter" is feeding well and settling. That's what matters.'

'Haven't you decided on the name yet?'

'No! Silly, isn't it? Haven't had time to talk to my husband and make a decision. We'll get there, I'm sure!'

Mrs Leadbetter was sitting in her spacious kitchen, and I couldn't help noticing there was a large pile of washing up in the sink, which was unusual in this normally immaculate home. The bin next to the back door was overflowing and the tiled floor looked like it could do with a sweep. This didn't worry me; in fact I was actually pleased she had not felt it necessary to keep up her high standards during these early days. I didn't want her to exhaust herself, and her priorities were to look after herself and the baby.

I asked Mrs Leadbetter if I could possibly use her telephone to respond to my bleep, and politely excused myself after I called the hospital and discovered that I had to go to a Mrs Potts in Hyde, whose waters had broken in the schoolyard earlier. She was now having strong contractions and did not feel she could make it to the hospital. The ambulance was on its way also.

Mrs Leadbetter seemed to brighten on hearing another baby was imminent, and wished me good luck. It could be quite awkward having to ask to make a call in someone else's house, as even in the early Nineties many people still viewed the telephone as an expensive device that was to be used as sparingly as possible. Only the day before, my request to use a phone in another home had been met with sideways glances, and I dialled the maternity unit number feeling quite awkward, promising to keep the call as brief as possible. Mrs Leadbetter was delighted to be of assistance, however, and I was grateful to her.

It was about eight miles from where I was in Glossop to Mrs Potts's house on Dowson Road in Hyde. The rush-hour had passed, and I expected the journey would take me about twenty minutes at the most. I hadn't banked on there being a heavy downpour just as I set out, however, and as I drove along Sandiway and Leicester Drive the rain bounced noisily off my car and seemed to make everyone drive at a snail's pace.

My windscreen wipers were going ten to the dozen as I sat at one red traffic light after another, seeing the clock on my dashboard tick away another minute, and another. A milk float had broken down on the Stockport Road, creating yet more of a hold-up, and I sat gripping the steering wheel anxiously as I waited my turn to steer past the drenched milk-man, who was desperately trying to cover boxes of eggs and glass bottles full of milk and orange juice with flimsy sheets of tarpaulin.

Finally, a full thirty minutes after leaving Mrs Leadbetter, I found Mrs Pott's address. There was an ambulance parked up outside the terraced house and I tucked my car up behind it and ran up to the front door, splashing my feet though puddles on the pavement as I did so.

An ambulanceman I'd never seen before threw open the door, took one look at me and shouted into the sitting room: 'The midwife's here!'

'She's in there,' he directed. 'She's had the baby. They both seem well.'

I pushed open the door to the sitting room, which was through a door immediately to my left, just off the small hall-way at the foot of the stairs. My adrenaline was flowing, because I knew that for a woman to deliver in the sitting room must have meant things had happened very quickly, or else she would have had the baby upstairs in her bedroom. In my mind's eye, I imagined poor Mrs Potts might be lying on the floor down here, waiting for me to deliver the placenta.

Ambulancemen are only given guidelines on how to deliver babies, and they do not deliver the placenta. That job is always left to the midwife, and in such cases the ambulanceman relies on the midwife to carry Syntometrine, the drug used to help facilitate the swift delivery of the placenta.

To my surprise, Mrs Potts was sitting up on the sofa cradling her baby in a fluffy green towel. The baby's cord was trailing out of the bottom of the towel and led to a red plastic bucket that was placed beside her on the settee. Inside the bucket was the placenta.

'Am I pleased to see you,' she smiled shyly. 'These two have been great but, can they go now?' She gave an embarrassed nod towards two burly ambulancemen who were standing like a couple of soldiers, guarding her on the settee.

'Yes,' I said, thinking how awful it must have been for her to have sat there like that, surrounded by men she had never met before, 'But I will just check you and the baby first, if I may, before they go.'

The placenta usually takes many minutes to separate from the wall of the uterus after the birth of the baby, and midwives usually give the injection of Syntometrine to hasten this separation and lessen any bleeding. In Mrs Potts's case nature had worked perfectly well, and as it had taken me thirty minutes to arrive I had actually allowed nature to do exactly what it should.

'Do you feel able to go upstairs?' I asked Mrs Potts. I wanted to check her and the baby over in the bedroom, where she would finally have the privacy she deserved. She nodded gratefully, thanking the ambulancemen as she got to her feet.

'I can't believe what just happened,' she said as we climbed the stairs together. 'I really can't.'

Once she was settled on the bed I checked Mrs Potts and her baby, cut the cord and made sure the placenta was complete before I nipped downstairs to thank the ambulancemen again before they left.

The baby was a pretty little girl with a fine head of hair that was so blonde it looked almost white. She had a bit of waxy vernix on her pale skin, probably down to the fact she was born a week early, but she appeared to be perfectly healthy.

'Do you know the chaos you've caused?!' I said gently to the baby as I examined her again thoroughly. 'Honestly, how can a little mite like you cause all this fuss for your mummy?!' I said it loud enough for Mrs Potts to hear, and when I looked up she was smiling, which is exactly the effect I wanted to have on her.

'All's well that ends well,' I told Mrs Potts as I set about examining her again. I needed to be sure her postnatal blood-loss was minimal, and was pleased to see that everything was absolutely as it should be.

'That's good,' she replied when I told her all was in order. 'I couldn't believe it when I wanted to push. The ambulance had literally just pulled up outside. I thought about trying to get up the stairs, but there was no way I would have made it. I only just managed to stagger to the front door to let the ambulance-men in. They were brilliant. Just brilliant. One of them fetched towels from the airing cupboard. He even made sure he covered the settee with the oldest looking ones …'

I stayed with Mrs Potts for a while, during which time she continued to talk and talk, often telling me the same thing over and over again. She also spoke to her mother and sister on the telephone and told them the whole story from start to finish, too. Her husband was driving home from a sales meeting in Glasgow, and he got a detailed description of the birth, too, when he called from a phone box at Charnock Richard Services on the M6.

It's very important for a woman to discuss her birth experience, particularly if it's been unusual, dramatic or alarming in any way. Nowadays we have specialist midwives who deal specifically with cases like this, where the woman is possibly traumatised by her delivery experience and may need to debrief. Often she just needs some reassurance that she has done nothing wrong, and that indeed all *is* well that ends well.

I have heard many stories of women who have threatened to complain or even sue the hospital when their birth has not panned out as they wanted it to, but in the vast majority of cases the woman decides not to complain after a day or two, when she has had time and space to talk and reflect on what actually happened.

When I left Mrs Potts that day I felt hopeful she would recover well from the shock of sharing the settee with her placenta. I checked on her every day until her baby girl, Jennifer, was ten days old, and was very pleased to see that Mrs Potts appeared to be really enjoying being a mother and was none the worse for her ordeal.

I often say that you are constantly surprised as a midwife, and the cases of Mrs Leadbetter and Mrs Potts remind me to this day how very true that is. Within the space of a few months I bumped into both women by chance, when they were no longer in my care. Mrs Leadbetter was pushing a pram around a supermarket in Glossop, and I saw Mrs Potts walking down a street in Hyde when I went to deliver another lady in the neighbourhood.

It turned out that, far from suffering any lasting upset or embarrassment as a result of her dramatic birth experience, Mrs Potts looked back on it with great amusement now, and had happily shared the story with all her friends and neighbours. 'I've got the best bucket collection in Hyde,' she told me brightly. 'Everyone thought the story was really funny, and lots of people bought me a new bucket as a joke. I've got half a dozen at least, in a variety of colours!'

Mrs Leadbetter, by contrast, had been through a rough patch a month or so after 'possibly Peter's' birth.

'Those baby blues came back,' she told me with a shrug when I asked how she'd been keeping. 'I did my best not to let them. Didn't want my husband to worry. But then I couldn't stop the tears any more.'

She went on to tell me that several weeks after she was discharged from our care she burst into tears in the library after realising she had brought the wrong books back for renewal.

'I cried all the way home and didn't stop for about four hours, until my husband came home and found me.'

The GP prescribed a short course of medication and advised Mrs Leadbetter to stop being so tough on herself. 'He was right,' she said. 'I can see that now. I was trying to be Mrs

Perfect and it was wearing me out. Once I realised I didn't have to be perfect all the time, I actually started to feel so much better.'

She gave me a big smile and pulled her shoulders back. 'I'm on the mend,' she said. 'Don't worry. I just never thought having a third baby would be so hard!'

Her chubby-cheeked little boy was sound asleep in the pram, and I asked her whether 'possibly Peter' was now just plain Peter. 'No,' she replied. 'He's David. Definitely David! You see – I even had to give myself a hard time over choosing the name. Typical!'

Postnatal depression was a medically recognised condition by this time, but it was nowhere near as well understood as it is today. I think it's true to say most people were a little wary of admitting to having it, for fear of being stuck with the stigma of suffering from a mental disorder, whereas nowadays it is freely talked about.

I do not remember Mrs Leadbetter using the term 'postnatal depression', and I'm sure I didn't, either, although she'd clearly had a dose of it. I have never forgotten her case, though, as in years to come I would be reminded time and time again that high-achieving women like Mrs Leadbetter can sometimes be more prone to suffering from postnatal depression than others. I can only speak from my own experience, but I have found that the more highly educated, aspirational and ambitious a woman is, the more pressure she puts herself under to be perfect in every aspect of her life, which can often lead to feelings of inadequacy and failure when those impossibly high targets are not met.

I will never forget how liberated Mrs Leadbetter looked that day when we said our goodbyes and she headed down the baby milk aisle. 'So much for the breastfeeding,' she smiled, reaching for a tin of formula. 'All I can say is I did my best. And thank the Lord for formula milk!'

'That's the spirit,' I thought. She'd done her best, and that is all any mother can do. Good for her.

'Hello! It's the midwife here!' I called. I'd been diverted from a home visit in Broadbottom to a big old farmhouse not too far away on Long Lane in Charlesworth. It was the summer of 1992 and I had a student midwife named Joanne with me.

Farmer's wife Nancy Stape had gone into spontaneous labour and called an ambulance, hoping she could be rushed to hospital in time to give birth there, which was her preference. However, it was standard practice for the ambulance crew to request a community midwife to also attend, just in case it was too late to make the dash to hospital. It was Mrs Stape's third baby, and at this point in time that was about as much as I knew. As she was not meant to be having a home birth, I'd never met her before.

'Hello! … Hello!' I called at the front gate, which was wedged tight shut even though the bolt across the inside of it was unlocked. I'd parked the car up behind the ambulance I'd spotted on the narrow lane running past the house and, when nobody answered my call from the gate, I began to struggle to try to open it, so Joanne and I could walk up the narrow pathway leading to the front door. The old property had acres of land around it and was surrounded by an old stone wall that was tumbling down in parts. The front garden was extremely muddy, else I might have suggested we should climb over part of the broken wall when our cries were not immediately answered.

'Hello!' I shouted, louder this time. I could see the front door was ajar, and was willing somebody to appear in the doorway. 'Can anybody hear me? It's the midwife here!'

Suddenly, Joanne grabbed my arm and screamed, and I looked up to see a big, fat pig with black patches on its enormous belly charging towards us. Before we knew it the hefty beast was pushing itself up against the gate, as if to tell us we were not welcome here.

Joanne stumbled backwards in alarm and slipped over, splattering mud all over her uniform, which unfortunately was a white dress. 'What are we going to do?' she asked as she picked herself up and looked at her dirty hands. I thought she was going to cry.

'We'll just have to barge our way through,' I replied. 'We're going to miss the delivery at this rate.' I could just imagine how Mrs Tattersall would have reacted in this situation. Cursing and frowning, she'd have been demanding to know how the 'ruddy hell' we were meant to go on now, and she might well have told Joanne to stop being a 'drama queen' and pull herself together. One thing was certain: Mrs Tattersall would not have been defeated.

'Right, we're going to have to just push together,' I said to Joanne. 'On the count of three … one, two, threeeeeeeee.'

It was no use. It seemed the harder we pushed at the gate, the more awkward the pig became, ramming himself up against the other side of it as if he were some kind of guard dog.

'Right, let's go again. Are you ready? One, two … oh, thank goodness!'

A giant of a man in green corduroy trousers that were belted beneath his large pot belly appeared in the front garden.

'Shoo you great oaf!' he shouted at the pig, before ramming it out of our way with impressive strength. 'Be off with you!' He continued to push the grunting pig until it was completely out of the way, before yanking open the gate and escorting us down the path to the house.

'Ever so sorry. That animal definitely thinks it's a guard dog, not a pig. Hope you've not been there long? Nancy's had the baby! Little boy. Lovely little fella. Come on up.'

Joanne and I exchanged glances. I think we were both disappointed to hear that after all our efforts to rush to Nancy's aid, we'd missed the big event, and I for one felt anxious about what I might find. Even though they always coped admirably, it wasn't ideal for the ambulance crew to deliver a baby, and I couldn't help an image of Mrs Potts sitting on the settee next to her placenta invading my thoughts as Joanne and I dashed upstairs to the master bedroom.

The scene that greeted us came as a very pleasant surprise. Nancy was sitting up and cradling her contented little boy in her arms, and there wasn't a paramedic in sight. The only other person in the room was a pretty little blonde lady whose face was glowing. 'Have you got any Syntometrine?' she asked. 'I'm Sharon Perkins. I'm a midwife at Stepping Hill. I live next door. Lucky I was in, hey? I normally go to aerobics when I'm off on a Tuesday.'

'Yes,' I replied with relief, taking the drug from my bag. I let Sharon deliver the placenta and we wrote up the notes between us while Joanne scrubbed her dirty hands and placed two plastic aprons over the front and back of her muddy dress.

'How are you feeling?' I asked Nancy.

'Absolutely fine,' she said to me. 'But what happened to *you*?' She was looking at the state of Joanne, who blushed and explained: 'It was the pig. He wouldn't let us in.'

Nancy cracked up laughing. 'Oooh, that hurts,' she chuckled, clutching her abdomen. 'Don't make me laugh again, please!' Kissing her son tenderly on the head, she said: 'Look at the trouble you've caused, turning up early. I don't know.'

It was one of those moments when everything in the world felt good. This mother's love for her child transcended absolutely everything, and it wouldn't have mattered if we were all covered in mud at that moment, because Mother Nature had worked her magic.

I discussed with Sharon that she would have to apply in retrospect to be allowed to practise in Glossop, as each midwife is only registered to work in certain areas and this was not one of hers. The paperwork would be a formality, however, and I was very pleased that things had worked out so well for Nancy.

Mr Stape made sure he escorted us back down the path when we left a couple of hours later, having enjoyed several cups of tea and some delicious home-baked scones. 'Don't worry,' he soothed. 'I've just filled the swill. That daft porker won't bother you now.' We told him we wouldn't have been bothered if we'd had to run the gauntlet of the pig all over again. All that really mattered was that our patient was safe and well and was now the very content mother of a gorgeous little boy.

Mr Stape gave Joanne and me a basket overflowing with fresh vegetables, and thanked us kindly. He'd done the same with the ambulance crew, who in the event had done nothing but had a cup of tea and a scone in the farmhouse kitchen, and waited until we arrived before heading to their next job. Goodness knows what Mr Snape gave Sharon as a thank you gift, as she certainly had been the key professional at the delivery. I placed the goodies in the boot of my car alongside Nancy's placenta, which was in a sealed container ready to be taken back to the hospital for disposal.

'Now there's a delivery we won't forget in a hurry,' I chuckled to Joanne as we pulled away, and we were still laughing when we arrived at the maternity unit some time later.

We decided to grab a cup of tea in the labour ward kitchen before we headed back out to do the four postnatal home visits we had planned that afternoon.

Joanne disappeared off to change her uniform while I put the kettle on, and I was very pleased when one of my colleagues, Sue, appeared. I hadn't seen her since I'd gone out into the community, and we had plenty to catch up on. Of course I told her the tale of the pig, which made her laugh, but I was very upset when she told me that unfortunately one of her recent deliveries had been memorable for very sad reasons.

'Linda, it was just awful,' she began. 'Honestly, just thinking about it makes me want to cry all over again.'

Sue went on to explain that one of her patients, a young Sri Lankan woman, had given birth to a baby with achondroplasia, a type of dwarfism. The genetic disorder had not been detected antenatally, as baby scans were nowhere near as detailed then as they are now, and as a result they did not pick up all the warning signs they would today. The mother was totally shocked when she saw her child, as it was immediately apparent that the baby had shortened limbs.

'It was one of those awful moments when everything goes very quiet in the delivery room,' Sue said. 'There was nothing.

Even the baby was silent, and then the mother started to sob and wail and completely broke down.'

The condition is extremely rare, occurring in approximately one in twenty-five thousand births. I had certainly never come across a case of it before, and I asked Sue how she dealt with it.

'I tried to reassure the mum that even though the baby didn't look as she expected, he was not actually ill. He was breathing normally, he was pink and his reflexes were good … I said as many positive things as I could, but she covered her face and refused to look at her baby, let alone take him in her arms. I said that the doctor would come and talk to her soon, but she told me she didn't want to see anyone. "Leave me alone and take that baby away," she said.'

I gave Sue a hug. 'You poor thing, that must have been absolutely dreadful to cope with. I can't imagine what that poor lady was thinking. How are things now?'

Sue shook her head. 'Not good. I've just spoken to Social Services. The mother has refused point blank to have anything to do with her baby. In fact, she has threatened to harm him if he is left in her care, and so Social Services have placed him with foster carers. It's out of our hands, but I can't get it out of my head.'

'Honestly, nature can be so very cruel,' I said. It was certainly not the first time I had used this phrase. The last time was just a month or two earlier when another colleague told me about a very sad case of a cot death. The three-week-old baby had died despite the mother following the latest advice to put babies to sleep on their backs. The television presenter Anne Diamond had fronted the 'Back to Sleep' campaign after her son Sebastian died from Sudden Infant Death Syndrome in

1991. In time we would learn that the campaign was a major success, with the number of cot deaths falling from more than two thousand a year to just three hundred, but of course it did not eliminate such tragedies altogether.

I never dealt directly with a mother who had lost her baby in a cot death, but when the occasional story reached the maternity unit there was always what I can only describe as a period of mourning, when midwives would talk quietly to each other, as if at a funeral.

Although I do not attend church regularly I still believe in God, despite encountering terribly sad cases like these and wondering why such things happen. I think my convent school education at Harrytown High School with Sister Mary Francis left me with an indelible faith that I believe has helped me in both my personal life and my work as a midwife. When times have been tough I've found it comforting to think there is a God up there, watching over us. Without God, perhaps life would be even harder?

I'm sure it would, and both my religious education and my work as a midwife have taught me that, though life can be terrible at times, there is always hope.

Chapter Thirteen

'Honestly, you could have been killed!'

'I'm Stacey and this is Shane. We fancy a water birth, we do.' Stacey was dressed in a short leather mini-skirt that was stretched across her tiny bump, fishnet tights, black Dr Marten boots and a leather jacket pitted with studs. Her hair was flamingo-pink and styled in a short, stiff Mohican. It was April 1995 and we were at an antenatal clinic in Glossop.

I invited the couple to sit down, which set off a lot of rattling of the chains that were hanging from Shane's leather jacket and drainpipe trousers. He had a very tall bleached blond Mohican with blue stripes running through it, and a T-shirt with 'The Sex Pistols' emblazoned across the front in red, white and blue.

'We've read up on water births and all that is involved, haven't we, Stace?' Shane said.

'Yes, we have. I think it'll be brilliant for me. I love being in the water, it will be so much better for me than being stuck in hospital. Shane's mam knows someone we can hire a pool off. It's a proper one, imported from America.'

I liked this young couple immediately. There was something very endearing about the fact they were already so far ahead in their planning when Stacey was only twelve weeks pregnant. I explained gently that should there be any complications we might have to reconsider, as labouring and giving birth in water was only suitable for the most straightforward of deliveries.

'We know,' they both nodded, squeezing each other's hands. 'We've read up on it. But we really want to give it a go, if we can.'

It was only a few years earlier, in the early Nineties, when water births first started to come into fashion in Britain. It would be several years before Tameside Hospital offered women having their baby in hospital the opportunity to use a birthing pool during their labour and delivery, but that didn't stop a minority of woman like Stacey from planning a water birth at home. I'd done a couple before, and it always took a fair bit of planning. For a start, the couple needed to take delivery of the pool and find a suitable place in the home for it at precisely the right time; just prior to the due date but not too early, otherwise hire charges might mount up and the pool could clutter up the home.

Some critics claimed the use of birthing pools increased the risk of infection to the newborn, but studies didn't back this up. I must admit the first time I saw a water birth, on a teaching video, I felt quite anxious because it was all so new to me. I was at a seminar, and I think the 'old school' midwife in me was perhaps a little wary and resistant to change. My initial reaction was that women had given birth for centuries without using birthing pools, and maybe we didn't need to change the natural way of things.

However, once I'd actually delivered my first 'water baby' to a down-to-earth primary school teacher in the back room of a very ordinary semi-detached house in Dukinfield, I never looked back. It was a real 'wow' moment seeing the baby emerge ever so calmly into the warm water, and now I fully supported water births, as long as that is what the woman felt was right for her.

If all goes to plan, the water soothes and calms the mother during labour and reduces the need for pain relief, making the experience less traumatic for both her and the baby. That's what I'd experienced at each of the water births I'd attended, and I'd seen that even if the mother simply used the pool to labour in and then delivered out of the water, the atmosphere was generally more relaxed and the babies less stressed than in many conventional births.

I got to know Stacey and Shane very well in the months leading up to the birth. They weren't married, but despite both only being in their early twenties they had been together for seven years, after meeting at school. Stacey worked part-time nights in a call centre and Shane helped his mate run a record shop near the viaduct in Stockport. Each time I saw them their excitement about becoming parents seemed to have increased ten times as much as Stacey's expanding abdomen.

When the call finally came that Stacey was in labour, I was absolutely delighted to be on duty. Even when both the community midwife and the patient dearly wished to be paired together, commitments with other patients, scheduled days off and annual leave meant it didn't always work out that way, so this was terrific timing.

Driving to their small terraced home, I felt very excited. We'd talked at length about how to prepare the pool correctly, and Stacey had told me she was going to choose some of her favourite music to play during the labour and birth. I'd spoken to Shane on the phone after he'd called the hospital with the news that Stacey was experiencing regular contractions that were becoming steadily stronger and closer together. He sounded really calm and told me proudly: 'The house looks amazing. We've got the pool in the middle of the front room and the atmosphere is wicked!'

'That's good,' I replied. 'I'm looking forward to seeing you. I'll be with you very shortly.'

It was exactly 6 p.m. when I stepped out of the car outside Stacey and Shane's house. To my surprise, I could hear thumping music coming from the front room and I had to knock loudly on the front door and the window several times before Shane finally let me in. He was dripping wet and had a skimpy towel draped around his narrow hips.

'Hi, Linda! Come on in! It's all happening!'

He was shouting to make himself heard above the music.

'Sorry it's a bit loud, but Stacey likes it like that. Hope you don't mind.'

'Well, perhaps it might be best to turn it down a little …'

I stopped in my tracks as I walked into the lounge. Stacey was squatting naked in the birthing pool, and there were strings of fairy lights draped all around the room. One set was dangling dangerously close to the water and looked as if it could dip into the pool any second.

I was horrified but tried to stay as calm as possible. 'Are those lights not a little too close to the water?' I said. 'I'm worried they could electrocute you. Where's the socket? Let's turn them off for a minute.'

'I'll do it,' Shane stammered.

'No, I'll do it. You're all wet.'

Moments later the panic was over after I'd switched off all the fairly lights at the wall and removed them from harm's way. I'd also got Shane to turn the music down, which he did reluctantly, explaining it was Stacey's favourite Sex Pistols track, 'God Save the Queen'.

'I wanted to be able to shout along to it, when the pains got worse,' Stacey said, looking a bit peeved.

'Well, let's just get ourselves sorted out first, shall we, before we start worrying about the music? Honestly, you could have been killed! You gave me a terrible shock. Could you not see the danger?'

I don't think I had ever spoken so sharply to a labouring woman or her partner before, but the shock of what might have happened really unnerved me, and I couldn't help giving the young couple a good talking to, once the risk was removed.

'Sorry about that. Is it OK if I get back in now?' Shane asked sheepishly when I'd said my peace and order appeared to have been restored.

As he spoke he stepped towards the pool and dropped his towel. I was completely shocked all over again, as he had nothing covering him except a tattoo on one buttock that said: 'Never Mind the Bollocks'.

'No, Shane, you cannot get back in the pool. Please cover yourself up at once. The pool is for Stacey, not you. For heaven's sake! What were you thinking?'

'But I was rubbing her back ...' he protested. 'What if I put a pair of shorts on?'

'No! You can sit on the side and rub her back.'

Stacey suddenly yelped in pain, and thankfully her timely contraction marked an end to the shenanigans and I could at last focus on assessing her progress and checking all was well with her labour, which thankfully it was. As I did so, Shane got dressed and put some sort of whale music on the stereo, which wasn't to my taste but seemed to soothe Stacey, and was a vast improvement on the blaring Sex Pistols racket.

When the light began to fade an hour or two later, Shane switched on the glaring main lights in the room. They didn't create the magical effect the couple had hoped for with the fairy lights, but at least they were safe, and that is the number-one priority during any birth.

Stacey got in and out of the pool once or twice during her fairly short labour, crouching over a beanbag and draping herself over the settee. Shifting into a variety of different positions certainly seemed to help her cope. When I think back to the early days of my career, when nobody ever considered that a woman might give birth in any other position than lying flat on her back, it still surprises me. Women like Stacey, who are prepared to push the boundaries, are the reason pregnant women today have so much say in their birth plans. It was always the women themselves who pushed for changes over the years, and midwives and the NHS responded to their wishes.

A second midwife arrived, which was standard practice, and I delivered Stacey's little girl at about 9 p.m. She was born on a duvet covered with towels on the floor of the lounge, after Stacey decided she didn't want to get back in the pool. She said she felt cold, and Shane gave her his ripped T-shirt with a skull on the front, which she was wearing when she gave birth. He was topless when the big moment came, which we all had a laugh about afterwards.

The little girl screamed blue murder when she was born, drowning out the whale music on the CD player, which had been left on 'repeat' and had played over and over again, giving me quite a headache.

Shane placed his arms protectively around Stacey and the baby and kissed them both tenderly. I can still picture them to this day. Shane's rebellious blond Mohican looked quite out of place in this scene of domestic bliss. Stacey's hair, though still shocking pink, was hanging down in damp waves around her face and she looked absolutely beautiful, her skin glowing and her make-up free eyes shining. Their daughter had tiny bubbles around her mouth and was incredibly fair and pretty. Stacey and Shane commented on how tiny her fingernails were, and marvelled at the softness of her pink, unblemished skin.

My colleague and I left the happy little family a couple of hours later, after Shane made us all a plate of scrambled eggs. The food was absolutely delicious, and I enjoyed it all the more as it was the very first time a new dad had ever cooked a meal for me. I had a very good feeling when I drove home that night. This pair really loved each other, and everything they had done, despite their mistake with the lights, was designed to make the birth of their baby extra-special, which it was.

Jonathan and Fiona were all ears later that night when I relayed the events of the evening. Jonathan was now twenty-one years old and Fiona was sixteen, going on seventeen. They had always shown a lot of interest in my job and loved hearing about my latest delivery, though neither of them ever expressed any wish to follow in my footsteps or work in a medical setting. Jonathan had always been very arty and by this time was doing a degree in Product Design at Huddersfield University, and was home for Easter.

Jonathan's art work was excellent, and once or twice I'd asked him to design me some posters for the parenting classes that I'd been teaching for several years, in the evenings. One particularly memorable poster, which he drew when he was studying for his A levels at Clarendon Sixth Form College in Hyde, depicted how a woman's facial expression changes during labour. He drew a whole series of images showing how smiles turn to frowns and then tears of pain.

Fiona, on the other hand, had her heart set on becoming an accountant, and was doing her A levels at Ashton Sixth Form College. Looking back, Fiona tells me that what she loved most about my job when she was growing up was that it meant the subjects of contraception and pregnancy were always openly discussed in our house, and if ever Fiona's friends needed advice or information she could generally provide it, after asking me first.

The three of us really enjoyed each other's company and shared some really good times. My mum used to say we were like the 'three Musketeers', as we made a great team together and always had lots of fun in the house in Stalybridge. Home was like a haven for me and I always enjoyed putting my key in the door after a long day at work.

I didn't tell Fiona and Jonathan everything about my work, of course, because some stories I felt were just too sad to bring home. Not long after Stacey's water birth, in fact, there was one such birth that sticks in my mind. I arrived at the maternity unit to collect some equipment in June 1995 to find one of my old colleagues, Annie, drying her eyes with a tissue on the corridor.

'Whatever's the matter?' I asked.

'It's Charlotte Cook. She had the baby tonight.'

My heart sank. I knew Charlotte's history, as it had been discussed by many midwives over the previous few months.

'How brave,' I think every single person who heard Charlotte's story said. 'What an amazing woman.'

When Charlotte had her routine blood test at sixteen weeks, it was discovered that her baby had a condition known as Potter's Syndrome, which is a severe chromosome abnormality. It was explained to Charlotte that her baby would not survive for more than perhaps a few hours after delivery, and very sadly she was offered a termination. Annie had been the midwife to break the awful news.

'No, thank you,' Charlotte had replied straightaway. 'The baby will die when it's ready to die, naturally.'

Charlotte was a lovely young lass who lived with her new husband in Dukinfield. They were not regular church-goers, but Charlotte had been educated by nuns in a convent school and had told Annie that her conscience could not have allowed her to go through with a termination.

'I can't explain it,' Charlotte had said to more than one midwife. 'I don't really see myself as religious, but this just feels right. I will carry the baby as long as I can, and fate will decide how long he or she lives.'

I remember Annie telling me all this, and I felt very moved. I had never been in such a dreadful situation myself, but I felt I could identify with Charlotte's reaction to her misfortune. Having also been educated by nuns, I still felt guided by their teaching, even all these years on. Sometimes, even today, I look up to the heavens and ask God what is the right thing to do, and I always follow my instincts, just as Charlotte did.

Annie cried as she told me she had delivered Charlotte's baby earlier this evening. Charlotte had gone into labour two weeks early, at thirty-eight weeks, and fortunately the baby was delivered quickly. Charlotte cuddled her little girl until she died peacefully in her arms three-quarters of an hour later.

Annie subsequently asked me if I would accompany her to the baby's funeral, as she didn't want to go alone, and I agreed.

'I can live with myself now,' Charlotte told us poignantly as we stood paying our respects in a windswept cemetery, after watching the smallest coffin I had ever seen being lowered into the ground. We both nodded, and she didn't need to say any more. Charlotte's words were incredibly encouraging to hear in such a bleak setting, but they didn't stop both Annie and I shedding a great deal of tears.

I never saw Charlotte again, although I later heard from Annie that she fell pregnant very quickly after-wards, and went on to deliver a healthy little boy within the year.

'She deserves every happiness,' I remember saying to Annie. 'I will never, ever forget her.'

Just a few weeks after the funeral I found myself in tears once more, this time on hearing an inspiring story from one of the community midwives, Cathy, who I bumped into in the office. There must have been about two or three members of staff taking a break at the same time, but you could have heard a pin drop as Cathy told her story.

'I had a terrible shock when I walked into the bedroom,' she said. 'There was the new mum, crying her eyes out, dropping big wet tears all over the baby's blanket as she rocked him in her arms.'

For those of us who didn't know the background, Cathy explained that her patient, a well-educated lady called Amanda Stubbs, had given birth to a baby with Downs Syndrome very recently. The condition had not been identified whilst she was pregnant, as she had declined screening. Also, because Amanda was only in her mid-thirties, she would probably not have been considered in a high-risk category, and therefore had not been encouraged to have the relevant tests.

Cathy told us that when she delivered the little boy at home she suspected straightaway that he might have Downs Syndrome. He had a shorter neck than usual and his eyes slanted upwards a little, but, most tellingly of all, he had a large, deep crease across the palm of each hand. An experienced midwife can recognise these signs, but they are not absolutely definitive and so Cathy said nothing, knowing that there was a chance she might be wrong and that tests would need to be carried out in the hospital.

Cathy explained that she had been bowled over by Amanda's reaction when she was finally told by the paediatrician, more than two weeks after his birth, that little Terence did indeed have Downs.

'She was absolutely amazing,' Cathy said. 'She didn't seem fazed at all. She and her husband said it didn't change a thing. They were thrilled to bits to be parents, and they loved Terence dearly. In fact: "This little baby is a gift to us" were Amanda's exact words to me.'

'I don't understand,' Betty the auxiliary said now, looking puzzled. 'Why the big tears today?'

'That's exactly what I asked Amanda,' Cathy replied. 'I had a horrible feeling that she was going to say she'd had a delayed reaction to Terence's condition … but it was nothing of the sort. Quite the opposite, in fact!'

'What, then?' another midwife asked. We were all intrigued, itching to hear the end of the story.

'Well, Amanda had just received more test results from the hospital. It turned out that Terence has a small hole in his heart and needs surgery. She was just so upset for *him*, worrying about the operation and the pain *he* might go through.'

We all let out a collective sigh. What a lovely women Amanda was, and what a lucky boy Terence was to have a mother who was clearly so besotted with him that she put his feelings first despite the turmoil she must have been going through herself.

'Some women are incredible, aren't they?' Betty said, straightening her apron and crunching on a custard cream.

'You can say that again,' I replied. 'Makes it all worthwhile when you hear things like that, doesn't it?'

I felt very humble after hearing about the experiences of both Charlotte and Amanda. As ever, encountering such moving stories made me hold my own family that little bit closer to my heart, knowing how very precious they were to me. Even though I'd been single for the longest time ever in my life, I felt very happy and fulfilled, because of my children.

Whenever we chatted about their careers and hopes and dreams for the future, I was always very keen for Jonathan and Fiona to follow their hearts and make their own decisions. When I looked at my brother John and myself, our paths could not have led in more different directions, with him still forging ahead very contentedly with his journalism career. We both enjoyed an enormous amount of job satisfaction, and I wanted the same for my children, and for my niece and nephew.

John's son Kerem was about to turn twenty-five and had decided to follow in his father's footsteps, which was entirely his choice. He had a job working for the Associated Press and was doing extremely well, living in London. I'd been lucky enough to see more of him in recent years, as he spent some time studying at Manchester University and would come over and have his tea with us, which was always a pleasure. He had a lovely girlfriend called Lisa who now lived with him, and his life seemed perfect. My niece Tijen had attended a dancing school in London and had now joined a small group of dancers travelling the world. Everybody, it seemed, was happy, and following their heart.

Though Jonathan and Fiona had no interest in following in *my* footsteps, they were usually the ones who encouraged me to tell stories about my job, rather than the other way around. I vividly remember the two of them roaring with laughter when I relayed the story of the 'barbecue birth' as I called it. This happened in the very hot August of 1995, when I was called out to the home of one of our local GPs in Glossop. He was hosting a barbecue for friends in his back garden, and one of his guests was a heavily pregnant lady called Annabelle Rolfe.

'Thank you ever so much for coming, Linda,' the GP stuttered when I arrived. 'One minute poor old Annabelle was helping my wife cook sausages on the barbecue and the next minute she just started saying she needed to push … I think the other guests expected me to swing into action, but I'm *so* glad you're here …'

He led me through a conservatory attached to the back of the house and into a huge garden. Several guests were gathered in a gazebo close to the conservatory, and I could see Annabelle and the GP's wife at the far end of the garden. Annabelle was lying on the ground, crying out in pain.

'It's all right, everybody,' the GP called as we passed the group of guests. 'The midwife's here! Everything will be all right now!'

I had to smile to myself. Here I was being swept across the lawn at the home of one of the most highly respected GPs in the area as if I were a guest of honour parading down a red carpet. It amused me that even someone like him thought the magic words 'the midwife's here' made everything instantly better. I was a midwife, not a miracle worker! It was a thought that crossed my mind on more than one occasion, and I always ardently hoped I would be able to live up to expectations.

Annabelle was having her second baby and had planned a hospital birth. 'Can't move. Too late. St-st-stay-ing here!' she told me. I dispatched the GP and his wife to fetch a blanket and towels and to take the guests inside. The garden was very long and nobody could see exactly what was going on, but it didn't seem right for the guests to be sipping Pimm's and eating hotdogs in such close proximity.

Within a couple of minutes I had removed Annabelle's underwear from beneath her expensive-looking Blooming Marvellous smock dress, and had seen that the baby's head was visible. Three pushes later and a noisy little girl plopped out perfectly onto a brand new Marks and Spencer beach towel. I wrapped her up immediately as, despite the blazing hot sun, she was no doubt crying partly in protest at being born into a gently blowing August breeze, which would come as quite a shock after leaving the warmth of her mother's tummy. The smell of burnt sausages in the air might also have disturbed her a bit, as she was born literally within a few yards of the abandoned barbecue!

'Bravo!' I heard the GP cheer after his wife popped down and then went inside to spread the good news. 'Congratulations, Annabelle. Congratulations, Linda!' he called. I heard a round of applause break out, and Annabelle laughed with relief as she cradled her daughter in the sunshine.

'Did the guests carry on with the BBQ?' Fiona asked when I told her the story for the first time.

'No, I don't think so,' I replied. 'But I think one or two might have had another stiff drink to get over the shock of it all!'

'Honestly, Mum, you've got such a crazy job,' Jonathan often said. 'But I love telling people you are a midwife.'

Chapter Fourteen

'Linda, I've got some terrible news'

At 8 a.m. on the morning of 2 May 1996 I received a call from a lady called Julie Bevins, whom I'd been looking after ante-natally. She was booked on the Domino scheme, which meant that I would visit her at home during her early labour, accompany her to hospital when she was established in labour, deliver her baby in hospital and come home from hospital with her about six hours later, all being well. This meant mothers like Julie received the same continuity of care as home birth patients, but with the peace of mind of having a hospital delivery, which is what many women wanted. I really like the system and we still use it today. It means we get to know the woman very well prior to the birth, which makes for less anxiety and uncertainty on the day of the delivery.

Julie was a care worker and this was her second baby, as she already had a little girl. When I arrived at her house in Hadfield and examined her, Julie was already six centimetres dilated and had her bag ready by the front door so we could dash straight to the hospital. It had taken me twice as long as it should have done to travel to her home because of the rush hour traffic, and at 8.30 a.m. I made the decision that we should call an ambulance to take us to the hospital as quickly as possible.

'Are you sure we'll get there?' Julie puffed.

'Of course we will!' I replied as I helped her into the ambulance soon afterwards.

Julie was experiencing strong contractions but she was coping really well and still managing to talk calmly as we set off on our short four-mile journey via Stalybridge to Ashton. Julie had a full four centimetres yet to go, and I was confident we'd have her safely on the labour ward well before she was ready to push. Normally this stage of labour, dilating from six centimetres to fully dilated at ten centimetres, takes a couple of hours. This would give us plenty of time to get to the maternity unit.

Julie told me that her daughter was being looked after by her grandma, and that her husband was following on in the car.

'That's good. Everything's under control,' I said.

'I want to PUSH!' Julie suddenly blurted out as we passed Mottram Moor, which was only about halfway into our journey.

'Right, then. Please try not to push, Julie. Take some big deep breaths for me. We're not far away from the hospital ...'

The ambulance made an abrupt turn and Julie grabbed her abdomen and cried out in pain. 'I have to push. I have to PUSH!' She was wearing leggings and a pair of knee-high boots, and I decided we should try to get them off her as quickly as possible, although this proved rather difficult as I was being thrown around a bit in the back of the speeding ambulance.

There was one ambulance driver in the back with us, and he started trying to pull off the leggings before we'd got the boots off.

Julie actually managed to laugh because it was all such a muddle, but I decided we needed to stop the ambulance.

'Stop! Can you stop, please?!' I shouted to the driver, and he pulled over immediately. I wasn't worried about being bounced around, but I was concerned that if this baby really was about to be born, which now looked very likely, I wouldn't be able to deliver it safely. We had stopped at a set of traffic lights on Acres Lane and the driver put the claxon on. I could hear cars driving around us as our siren rang out and hazards flashed. I whipped off Julie's boots, leggings and underwear as fast as I could and saw the baby's head advancing.

'You are going to have the baby here in the ambulance, but everything is fine. Just do as I say and keep breathing. You are doing really, really well.'

I could hear noisy car exhausts and the sound of tyres on Tarmac, but instead of the smell of fumes and warm rubber I typically associated with the rush hour, my nostrils were filled with the sterile smell of hospitals. We most certainly weren't at the maternity unit, though, however familiar the smells were, and it was quite disconcerting to be delivering a baby in the middle of a busy road, albeit in the back of an ambulance.

'I don't believe this …' Julie groaned.

'Don't worry. It's fine. Can you just give me a very big push when I say so? Right, wait a bit, there you are. Push now, Julie!'

She was absolutely brilliant, gritting her teeth and following my instructions to the letter. Just a few pushes later she gave birth to a perfect baby boy. I wrapped him up in a blanket and tucked him down the jacket Julie was still wearing, to keep him warm.

'Thank you!' I called to the driver. 'You can carry on now and take us to the hospital! I shall deliver the placenta when we get there.'

'Will do. Congratulations!' came the reply, and we drove steadily to the hospital.

Julie looked ecstatic as she kissed her little boy's forehead. He was a good weight, very alert and was wriggling and having a little cry just as a newborn should. It warmed my heart to see mother and son looking so contented and bonded just moments after such a dramatic birth.

'I am going to call him Ayrton, after Ayrton Senna,' Julie told me later, and she did. I am pleased to say we are still in touch to this day, as Julie is a good friend of a nurse I know. Julie was also my father's carer months before he died in August 2009, at the age of 95, which was a great comfort for me.

It took quite a few years for us to be able to see each other *without* mentioning the ambulance, as it inevitably had a big impact on both of us, but we always agreed that, as unlikely as this may seem, it was a lovely experience.

Several months later, in January 1997, Tameside Hospital's maternity unit celebrated its official twenty-fifth anniversary. The *Coronation Street* actor Bill Tarmey, who played Jack Duckworth, made an appearance to mark the occasion, and some of the first babies born at the unit gathered to cut a cake and pose for the local press. Amongst them was a tall and handsome young man named Jarrod Randle. He attended with his mother Kathleen, who looked just as proud as she had in December 1971, when she had the honour of becoming the first mum ever to have her baby in the newly opened unit, several weeks before it was officially declared open at the start of 1972.

I remember letting off balloons in the car park on the day of the anniversary, wearing my navy blue midwife dress and red belt, enjoying the celebrations with colleagues. I was forty-eight years old, yet it really didn't seem possible that twenty-five years had passed since I'd excitedly witnessed the building of the new unit as a newly qualified midwife.

So many things had changed, and yet so many things had not. Just six months earlier, in June 1996, a huge IRA bomb went off in the centre of Manchester, injuring more than two hundred people and devastating the heart of the city I once knew so well, rendering some parts of it completely unrecognisable to me. Would the IRA ever stop? I'd known bombings all through my adult life, and the Troubles never failed to depress me.

Charles and Di got divorced that same year, and it was also the sixteenth anniversary of the death of John Lennon. I caught part of a documentary about his life on the radio, and was astonished that so many years had passed since he was shot in 1980. I'd been such a huge Beatles fan in my youth, but I'd grown up a lot since then. I was a mature woman now, not a teenager, and my days of screaming along to the Beatles felt a million years away.

So many things had altered in my personal life and in the world around me, although of course one thing had always stayed the same. I was happy in my job at Tameside. It had been a constant force for good in my life, despite the maternity unit going through many changes itself.

By this point in time, what was known as 'Changing Childbirth' was well established. This was a Government initiative introduced in 1993, with the aim of putting the wishes of mothers at the forefront of maternity care. I had seen with my own eyes how the women themselves had pushed for such changes to happen. Ever since the late Seventies, when women started to refuse routine shaves and enemas, change had been in the air, with women starting to voice their opinions in the maternity unit. In the Eighties many more began to speak out, querying whether or not they needed an episiotomy or a hospital birth, and asking many questions of doctors and midwives instead of simply being told what to do.

By the Nineties, when so much more information became available and the Internet entered the homes of ordinary people, it was time for action. Now we were in an era where women were encouraged to make a birth plan, choose from a range of different methods of pain relief, have a say in their antenatal care and decide where and how they would give birth. As midwives we welcomed Changing Childbirth with open arms. I believe every woman has the right to make her own decisions about the birth of her baby, and in my experience women are far happier when they feel in control of their pregnancy and delivery. You only had to look at the case of Stacey and Shane to see that, and I simply cannot imagine how they would have got on had they been told what to do every step of the way.

However, there was one change that I didn't welcome, and this was the arrival of the so-called 'compensation culture'. I have always made sure my practice is as safe as possible, which is all any midwife can do, but nevertheless it became harder over the years to ignore what has become an omnipresent threat: that a patient might sue. The vast majority of patients would not dream of taking legal action, but the difference was that by the Nineties midwives were very aware of what was *possible*, and I for one was extremely conscious of eliminating any risks whatsoever, which inevitably took some of the fun out of the job.

In the early Seventies I can remember on more than one occasion having patients who could see how busy we were saying jokey things to us like: 'Is it all right to push, Nurse, or are you on your break?'

I'd sometimes reply by saying: 'No, you can't as I've not had my cornflakes yet!' Of course, I had my tongue firmly planted in my cheek. We'd all laugh, knowing it was just light-hearted banter and there was no way in the world I would prioritise my breakfast over the needs of a patient. However, it was around the mid- to late-Eighties that I first recall becoming more cautious about what I said, in case a conversation might be misconstrued. Nowadays, I am more aware than ever of the threat of litigation, and it is always at the forefront rather than the back of my mind, which saddens me.

Of course, some grievances and complaints were genuine, as NHS care was not always faultless, as the extreme case of Harold Shipman was about to highlight. It was 1998 when he was first questioned about the high death rate among his patients.

'Not Fred!' was my immediate reaction. Colleagues who knew him, both professionally and personally, all said the same thing. 'Surely not Fred. It can't be true.' We all knew him as a caring, diligent GP and devoted family man. The news that he was even being questioned came as a shock, but I was sure there had to be some reasonable explanation, and that he couldn't possibly be at fault.

Fortunately, I also remember 1998 for another, much happier, reason. It was the year I met my late husband Peter, who I went on to marry in December 2000. I bumped into Peter in the chilled food aisle at Tesco in Glossop one warm afternoon in May. I was reaching for a pint of milk when I spotted him pushing his trolley towards me, and I instantly recognised him as an old friend of Ian's. I hadn't seen Peter for many years, but I knew that his wife had died and I told him I had been very sorry to hear that.

He smiled and thanked me for my kind words, and I was surprised when he told me that his wife had died several years earlier, a short time after I had split up with Ian, in fact. 'Goodness me, don't the years speed by?' I said.

'Indeed they do. Do you fancy going for a drink, to catch up on old times?'

I didn't hesitate in accepting, and was pleased when Peter suggested that it would perhaps be better to go for a meal instead, as he didn't really like just going out for drinks. I was happy to agree. We swapped numbers and arranged to go out the following Friday evening to a local restaurant called the Gunn Inn in Hollingworth. I found myself really looking forward to it, and I had a picture of Peter in my mind on and off all week. He was tall and looked rather distinguished with his silver-grey hair, but what I liked most about him was that he appeared to be the perfect gentleman. He always had lots to say and was always polite, qualities I admire.

I remembered that Peter worked as an electrician, and he knew I worked as a midwife, which was just as well, because I had forgotten I was on call, and in the late afternoon of the day we'd arranged to meet I had to attend a home delivery, and was forced to cancel our date.

'I'm really sorry, I'll probably be out all night, we'll have to do it another time,' I told Peter hastily.

'Not to worry,' he replied.

Peter told me later that he thought I'd changed my mind and didn't want to meet him, as I sounded very matter-of-fact. I can understand that, looking back, but nothing could have been further from the truth. I was simply focused on my patient, as she had to come first. I was really disappointed to have had to cancel, and when a week or so passed without Peter phoning me again as I'd hoped he would, I contacted him and rearranged the meal. I'm so glad I did. We really clicked, and chatted away very comfortably.

'How did the delivery go last week?' he asked.

'Fine, in the end,' I told him. 'But I nearly didn't get there.'

'Why? Were you going to come out with me after all?'

'No! I would never do that to a patient! You won't believe this, but the lady lived in Tintwistle, and the lane leading up to her house was blocked by half a dozen cows.'

'What did you do?'

'Well, I just had to sit tight for five minutes until they got bored of looking at me and decided to move on. What else could I do?'

Peter laughed his head off, and so did I. We didn't realise it then, but he and I would spend thirteen very happy years together, until his death in 2011. Jonathan and Fiona liked him very much, and as they became increasingly independent, I spent more time with Peter, thoroughly enjoying his company.

There were many more changes happening in my working life, too. By 1999, Betty had retired from midwifery and Carol had left to go to Ghana with her husband. Team midwifery was being introduced, which meant we would no longer be known as community midwives but 'team midwives', and would work both in the hospital and in the community. This change caused an awful lot of upset amongst many older midwives, and many felt very anxious about the change, myself included. I thought things were fine the way they were, and of course I'd already had to deal with Betty and Carol leaving, both of whom I missed very much.

It was at this time that I started to work with Helen Howard, who was to be my partner in our new team of five. The first day we met was in a staff room at the maternity unit, and I was quite taken aback as I felt an instant connection to her. It took me a few minutes to realise why, and then it dawned on me: Helen reminded me of a younger version of myself. Indeed, in my eyes she *was* a younger version of me. I was fifty-one years old and she was twenty years younger. I had come face to face with my thirty-year-old self; that's exactly how it felt. Straight-away I felt sure we would get on famously, and we did, right from day one. I helped Helen in her community work, and she helped me to readjust to working back in the hospital.

There was a lot of new equipment to familiarise myself with, such as hospital monitors which had become much more high tech, but by far the biggest change I had to contend with was in the increased use of epidurals.

'In the Eighties, you could only have an epidural if you came in between 9 a.m. and 5 p.m.,' I told Helen, explaining that only senior anaesthetists could perform them, and those were their working hours.

'I don't think women would accept that nowadays,' Helen laughed, explaining that epidurals were now extremely popular and in demand twenty-four hours a day. She talked me through how to assist the anaesthetist in setting up the equipment, and how to maintain the epidural by topping up the Lignocaine, which is the painkilling drug injected around the nerves in the small of the back.

'What's the secret to being a good community midwife?' Helen asked me in return.

'Well, it's certainly not just about delivering babies,' I said. 'Of course, that's the icing on the cake for any midwife, but there's a lot more to it than that.'

This is so true. I'd been in the community for eight years now, and I'd learned that the hours of antenatal care given to each and every pregnant woman were equally as important as the time spent reassuring them, showing an interest and sharing general chitchat with them and their partner. This also follows on into the delivery and postnatal period.

'The patients usually start off saying "the midwife's here" and end up saying "Linda's here,"' I explained to Helen. 'It will happen to you. The trust and confidence my patients have in me is almost tangible. I feel it in their smiles. I am so welcomed into their homes. They treat me like a member of the family. It's wonderful.'

Helen was all ears, and I was enjoying sharing my experience. She could have been *me*, so many years earlier, listening to Mrs Tattersall explaining how she might offer a high chair that was no longer needed in one household to a needy couple down the road, or suggest that a little sibling who was scratching his head might benefit from the head lice treatment she happened to have in her bag.

'But doesn't it take years of experience to build up that confidence and rapport with the patients?' Helen asked. 'Do you think the patients might be less trusting of me as I'm new in the community?'

'Not at all! You are sharing a very special time in a patient's life, and that is very bonding. I have to introduce myself to new mums all the time, and many have no idea how long I've been practising. If you enjoy your work, the patient can see that and you'll be welcomed with open arms. It'll be "Helen's here!" before you know it.'

Helen hung on my every word, and I knew she was going to be a terrific team midwife, because I could see she had a genuine passion for the job, and that is the best foundation any midwife can have.

As the year 2000 dawned, the maternity unit inevitably found itself in the spotlight. We were used to the local press turning up on 1 January to photograph the first baby born each New Year, but the advent of the new millennium had whipped the media up into quite a frenzy. I heard from colleagues that reporters from up and down the country had been in touch with our communications department, asking questions about the number of pregnant women who were in our care, who were likely to be in the running to deliver the UK's first millennium baby.

'What a lot of codswallop,' Jean, one of the auxiliaries, said. 'Surely you don't have to be a midwife to know that when it comes to babies being born, nothing short of a crystal ball can help you out there!'

I had to agree with her. I understood why the first new baby would make headline news, but I'd lost track of the number of silly conversations I'd had with people over the previous nine months or so on this subject.

'What date would I have to have got pregnant on to have a New Year's Day baby?' several women had asked me at the antenatal clinic over the past six months. 'Imagine that as your date of birth – 1 January 2000!'

None of the women made reference to the fact that the first millennium baby born in Britain would no doubt be showered with a whole lot more than mere publicity. The newspapers had been full of stories about the freebies that might be offered to the baby who claimed the title, and I was not the only midwife who suspected that this is what motivated some women to make a determined effort to fall pregnant exactly nine months before the New Year.

'Nobody would ever forget your child's birthday, that's for sure,' I always smiled whenever women brought up this subject. 'But please don't get hung up about the date. Honestly, enjoy your pregnancy and let fate take its course. Let Mother Nature decide.'

In the event, Tameside Hospital didn't get much of a look-in when the big day dawned, as many babies had already been born up and down the country by the time our first arrival was delivered.

Unfortunately, the entire Tameside region had been receiving a lot of publicity for another reason in recent months, as the trial of Harold Shipman had been going on since October 1999. He was charged with the murders of fifteen women, all of whom had died between 1995 and 1998. Journalists appeared to leave no stone unturned as they carried out background research prior to the trial, and Shipman's links with Tameside Hospital through his local GP practice were well known. I could scarcely believe my eyes or ears whenever I caught a news report on television or glimpsed an article referring to Tameside Hospital in the same sentence as 'alleged murderer Harold Shipman'.

Everybody I knew outside of work seemed to ask me the same question. 'You worked with him, Linda. You knew him. Do you think he's guilty?'

Every single time without fail I replied: 'No, I just can't believe it. There must be a mistake. Fred was such a nice man, the type who wouldn't harm a fly.'

My colleagues within the hospital, who all knew him as Fred, shared my disbelief. It seemed impossible that such a caring GP, the type of man who would arrive on the maternity ward in the middle of the night to offer support to one of his patients when he was not obliged to do so, could possibly be capable of murder.

On 31 January 2000 Shipman was found guilty of killing all fifteen patients by lethal injections of diamorphine, and of forging the will of one of the women, Kathleen Grundy. It had been the suspicions raised by Mrs Grundy's daughter over the authenticity of the will that had led to Shipman's arrest in September 1998, and prompted the wider investigation into other deaths he had certified.

I had just finished running an antenatal clinic when I heard the news of the guilty verdict. My head swam. I think I listened to the details on the radio, and I had to sit down. I thought about the time I had taken Fiona to Shipman's home, and how I'd drunk tea in his kitchen with his wife Primrose. I clearly saw myself lifting tables with him at the school fête, setting ourselves up together as willing first-aiders. I thought he was a pillar of the community, but all along I was rubbing shoulders with a mass-murderer.

It didn't seem real at all. I felt nauseous and I wanted to be physically sick, in fact. Don't get me wrong. I didn't think I, Fiona or, indeed, any of my patients had had a lucky escape from his clutches. From what I'd heard of the court case, it seemed clear that the majority of Shipman's victims fitted a similar mould, in that they were elderly and vulnerable and, in his view, no longer worth treating. For reasons we will never know, he chose to kill them, not care for them.

It really didn't seem possible, and I had several long conversations with Peter around this time, trying to make sense of it all. I always failed, and Shipman refused to give any hint of a motive for his crimes right up until the day he hanged himself three years later. By then the Shipman Inquiry had concluded that he was probably responsible for two hundred and fifteen deaths between 1975 and 1998. This made him Britain's worst serial killer, and the press dubbed him 'Dr Death'. It was such a shock, it really was.

I was very pleased that in the months after Shipman's conviction I had three far more positive events to concentrate on. Peter and I had set a date in December 2000 for our wedding, and in the October my nephew Kerem announced he was going to be married to his girlfriend Elida, a Kosovo Albanian. He had finished with his long-term girlfriend Lisa some time before, and had met Elida whilst working in Pristina in Kosovo, where they were both journalists for the Associated Press. They were also to be married in December, the week before Peter and me.

Shortly before their wedding, Kerem and Elida came to visit us and announced that Elida was fourteen weeks pregnant. I was so thrilled. This was the first time I had met Elida, but I warmed to her immediately.

'Have you heard the baby's heartbeat?' I asked.

'No, not yet.'

'Would you like to?'

She was so excited, and I shall never forget the look of absolute delight on Kerem's face as we all listened with my Sonicaid and heard the faint heartbeat.

'That's amazing!' he beamed, and my heart was full of love for him. Kerem was never afraid to show his feelings, and I thought Elida was such a lucky girl to have him as her partner.

On 15 December 2000, Kerem and Elida were married in Pristina, and on 21 December 2000, Peter and I tied the knot at Dukinfield Register Office. I was now Mrs Linda Sutcliffe, and I was extremely happy. We had a reception at home attended by a small group of family and friends, including my parents, of course, who by then were both in their eighties. 'I'm so pleased for you Linda,' Mum said. 'Are you going to change your name for work?'

Mum never altered a bit. It was typical of her to ask such a practical question, although I was also touched that she still cared about my working life, even after all these years. She had supported me throughout my career, and she had never stopped being interested and asking me questions about my job.

'Actually, I'm going to stay as Linda Fairley,' I told her, explaining that it hardly seemed worth the bother of changing my name at work, when I'd been known as Linda Fairley for twenty-odd years.

Dad smiled and nodded and sipped a glass of champagne. He was still a man who 'didn't want to be on the front row' as my mother always said. I was very fortunate to have them as my parents. I think they were probably as surprised as I was that I had married for the third time. Of all the things in my life, it wasn't something I was particularly proud of, although when I looked at Jonathan and Fiona that day, both wonderful children, doing well in their separate fields, I had no regrets whatsoever. Graham was still involved in Jonathan's life and, although he had moved away, Ian had always stayed in touch with Fiona.

I moved into Peter's house in Mottram. It is the home I still live in today, and I have nothing but fond memories of Peter all around me. He was a thoroughly kind and decent man, and he loved me and looked after me really well throughout our years together.

Tragically, just three months after our marriage, I needed a great deal of support from Peter after I received the most devastating news from my brother. It was 5.30 p.m. on 29 March 2001 when the phone rang in the sitting room at home.

'Hi, Linda,' I heard my brother's voice say.

'Hi, John,' I light-heartedly replied, pleased to hear him call.

'Linda, I've got some terrible news. Kerem has been killed in Kosovo,' he said. 'Go and tell Mum and Dad before they see it on the six o'clock news on television.'

My heart stopped. I can't remember what I said, but I know I put the telephone down and stared into space for a moment. We all loved my nephew so very much. He was thirty years old and was about to become a father. How could this possibly have happened? How must my brother and sister-in-law be feeling, and how would I tell my parents this dreadful news? As for myself, I could only think of Kerem's beautiful, smiling face when he heard his baby's heartbeat, here in my house, such a short time ago.

My dad had had an eye operation and couldn't see anything, and it was unbearably sad having to deliver such devastating news to both of my parents at this time in their lives. When I broke the news it was like someone had turned a light out; it was simply heart-breaking. Tijen, my niece, phoned to say she was going to Kosovo and would keep us informed, and when Peter got home from work I had to tell him also, and he was terribly upset. I hated seeing the people I loved suffering, but Peter seemed to know just what to say. I felt very comforted by him, and over the coming months and years he offered me no end of support.

Kerem had been based in Pristina, the capital of the Kosovo province, for several months and Elida was twenty-seven years old and twenty-eight weeks pregnant with their first child when he was killed. It happened when his car was hit by mortar shells in the Kosovan village of Krivenik, less than a mile from the Macedonian border.

He is listed on the Associated Press's 'Wall of Honor' of fallen journalists, which I have reproduced here, as it is such a moving and fitting tribute to my much-missed nephew.

KEREM LAWTON (1970–2001)

APTN producer Kerem Lawton was killed March 29, 2001, when his car was hit by mortar fire near the volatile Kosovo-Macedonian border. He was 30. Lawton was the husband of APTN producer Elida Ramadani. Born in Brussels, Belgium and raised in England, Lawton was the son of a Turkish mother and a British father. Bilingual in Turkish and English, he also spoke German, French and some Italian. Lawton joined the AP as a newsman in Rome and later joined APTN in Turkey. He immersed himself in assignments that sent him into the grimmest of circumstances – the conflict in Kosovo, the Kurdish insurgency in southeast Turkey, Albania's 1997 plunge into near-anarchy, ethnic tensions in China's Xinjiang province. Yet through it all, there was a sense of generosity about him, an infectious sense of fun. 'I do not exaggerate in saying that he was everyone's golden boy,' said Rome Chief of Bureau Dennis Redmont, a family friend. 'He had a lightness in a profession where many people are heavy hitters. Everyone wanted Kerem as his brother, his boyfriend and his son.'

Kerem was buried in Kew Gardens, and on 25 June 2001, Tara Kerem Lawton was born in London. Elida had a very difficult birth; she was still grieving so much. It was such a very sad time for us as a family, but Tara was a healthy and beautiful little girl, who made us smile again. John and Nevim adored her, and so did I. Tara is eleven years old now, and is still a lovely bright light in our family.

Chapter Fifteen

'It wasn't how I'd envisaged the birth at all!'

In the spring of 2001 I was running an antenatal clinic in Hollingworth one afternoon when a new patient called Julie came for her 'booking in' appointment. She was having her first baby and told me she was very much looking forward to becoming a mum. I liked Julie immediately. She was very smiley and down to earth, and didn't bat an eyelid when I ran through the usual battery of questions I was required to ask every new patient.

One or two women, typically the most well-to-do of my pregnant ladies, raised an eyebrow or said sniffily: 'Is this really necessary?' when I had to ask them if they had ever been a drug user, or had any of the risk factors for HIV. I would have to explain that, yes, I was obliged to ask such questions and that the information would be treated in the strictest of confidence, with the specific aim of safeguarding the health of both mother and baby. Julie, however, was extremely easy-going and took it all in her stride. 'Not much fazes me,' she giggled. 'That's good,' I replied.

The second time we met, Julie was just as pleasant, asking me about my own family and chatting about everything from maternity leave to breastfeeding. She told me she hoped to have a home birth, and asked me about the possibility I might be able to deliver her in October, when her baby was due. 'I'd like that very much,' I said. 'It's very difficult to guarantee I'll be available, but if I'm on duty I will do my very best.'

When my next patient, Zoe, came in she was grinning from ear to ear. 'I can't believe Hayley's in here!' she laughed. 'Fancy that!'

It had been many years since I'd watched *Coronation Street*, but Zoe was more than happy to tell me that Julie was none other than the famous Corrie actress Julie Hesmondhalgh, aka Hayley Cropper. 'I bet you had a right laugh!' Zoe said. When I looked at her bit blankly she went on to explain that the character Julie played was a transsexual, and that the character Hayley used to be a man called Harold. Julie's remark about nothing fazing her suddenly took on a sharper meaning, and I smiled to myself. No doubt she had been prepared for some jokey reference to her character's complicated biology, but of course none was forthcoming from me as I didn't even realise she was a well-known actress.

On Julie's next appointment I apologised for not having recognised her, explaining that my job meant it was quite diffi-cult to keep up with television soaps.

'I'm really sorry,' I said. 'I seem to be the only person around here who doesn't recognise you.'

'Actually, I was really pleased when you didn't,' she said. 'There's no need to apologise at all!'

I think that would have been the last word on the matter if I hadn't made an embarrassing slip-up on Julie's next visit. Scanning my appointment list for the next patient and seeing the name Julie Hesmondhalgh clearly written in black and white, I looked up hurriedly and called across the waiting room: 'Hayley, please!'

There was a momentary pause before Julie cracked up laughing and followed me into the antenatal surgery, leaving several other patients giggling in her wake.

'I'm so sorry!' I said, 'Really I am. I can't believe I've got to apologise to you again!'

'Honestly, it doesn't matter at all,' Julie said genuinely. 'Even my dad calls me Hayley sometimes. I'm not worried at all.'

We discussed the possibility of Julie having not only a home delivery but potentially a home water birth, and she went away to make enquiries about hiring a pool. 'I'm sure when I'm giving birth I won't mind what anybody calls me. As long as you're my midwife, I'll be fine, I'm sure.'

I was flattered, just as I had been when my colleague Helen had asked me if I would be *her* midwife when she had her first child in August 2001.

'I would love to, but are you sure?' I'd said, slightly hesitantly.

'Linda, there's nobody I'd like to deliver my baby more than you,' Helen told me.

'Well then, it'll be an honour.'

I got a call at 3 a.m. on 8 August to say Helen had gone into labour. We'd become like soulmates right from the word go, and I'd felt slightly daunted as her due date approached, hoping everything would run smoothly for her. Now I felt decidedly nervous. Helen was not just a colleague but one of my best friends, and I wondered if this was a good idea after all. Fortunately, as soon as I arrived at her house I had my answer, because I found myself automatically switching into professional midwife mode.

'You're doing well but I think you can stay at home for several more hours,' I told her, and I returned at 7 a.m. to find

Helen was six centimetres dilated, just as I'd hoped and expected.

She wanted to have her first baby at Tameside Hospital, and once we got her onto the labour ward she progressed really well. I administered Pethidine and talked Helen through her contractions just as I would any other patient, and she followed my guidance without questioning me. The added pressure I feared our friendship might put on the delivery just wasn't there, and in fact the atmosphere was very calm.

Angela, another Glossop team member, also arrived, and she was a huge support for me, telling me I was doing a good job and reassuring me, just as I was trying to do for Helen.

When William Henry Howard finally arrived he was the spitting image of his dad Dean, who looked very emotional as he witnessed the birth. I don't think I have ever heard so many congratulations being passed in every direction, all around the delivery room. I was delighted everything had gone to plan, and I am indeed very honoured to have been at the heart of such a wonderful event in my friend's life.

A couple of months later it was Julie Hesmondhalgh's turn to have her baby. We'd discussed her plans to have a water birth and I knew Julie had the birthing pool ready and waiting at her home. Unfortunately, as is often the case in midwifery, the very best-laid plans sometimes have to be cast aside. When I visited Julie at her home as her due date approached, I found that her waters had broken, but her labour wasn't progressing.

Ultimately, Julie had to go into hospital to be induced, which meant that not only was her planned water birth not possible, but I did not get to deliver her. This outcome could not have been more different to the one she had hoped for, but

Julie was typically magnanimous and gave me a broad smile when I popped in to see her and the baby in a side room at the maternity unit on 14 October 2001.

'The staff were wonderful and looked after me really well,' she said as she proudly showed off her very pretty day-old daughter. 'It was fine, Linda, honestly.'

After being induced, Julie had to deal with the further complication that her daughter's cord was wrapped round her neck, which resulted in Julie requiring an emergency Caesarean.

'It was very strange coming round from the anaesthetic and being handed my daughter,' Julie said. 'Needless to say, it wasn't how I'd envisaged the birth at all!'

As with the majority of new mothers, once their newborn baby is safely in their arms, the unexpected twists and turns of the delivery are forgotten. Julie was certainly one of those mums, and her focus was all on her precious baby, who weighed in at ten pounds, eight ounces and was named Martha Mo.

Once she was back home I visited Julie every day for ten days. We would sit on a bench in her kitchen and chat about everything under the sun. It was always a pleasure to visit Julie because she was such a positive, warm person. She never complained about anything, and had nothing but good things to say about the care she had received.

On my way home from seeing Julie one day I called in to see a lady called Kimberley, who lived nearby and was a friend of one of my other patients.

'She's recently had a miscarriage,' my patient had told me. 'And she didn't see a midwife because she miscarried so early.

I've told her all about you, and she said she'd love to speak to you.'

I was happy to call in for a cup of tea and a chat, if it might help Kimberley, and I'm very glad I did.

'I've heard your name mentioned so many times by different friends,' Kimberley told me as she brewed a pot of tea and offered me a piece of shortbread. 'I just wanted to tell you my story, to see what you think.'

I told her that of course I was willing to listen, and I found myself being very moved by what Kimberley told me.

'We've been trying for a baby for nine years,' she explained. 'I finally got pregnant on the second attempt at IVF, but I miscarried after just three weeks.'

I let Kimberley tell me as much as she wanted to about the difficulties she'd had over the years, and was very upset to hear how much she had suffered with the painful IVF process, not to mention how much she and her husband Duncan had sacrificed to find the money for the treatment.

'What do you think I should do now, Linda?' she asked, her eyes searching my face for the answer to her prayers.

I was very careful not to offer any specific advice, or to say anything that might give false hope. A woman who has suffered a miscarriage does not want you to tell her it will all be fine next time because she knows well that nobody can say that.

'What do *you* think you should do?' I asked.

'I want to try again, definitely,' she said. 'I don't want to give up.'

I gave her a smile and told her if she felt that way, she should follow her heart.

'Perhaps give yourself a little bit of breathing space first,' was all I said. 'But if that's how you, and your husband, are feeling, and the doctors are happy for you to try again, I think perhaps you should.'

I saw Kimberley a few months later, by chance, on the High Street in Glossop.

'You helped me so much,' she told me. 'I honestly couldn't think straight, but you just let me talk and come to my own conclusion. We're going to try one last time with IVF. Thank you, Linda.'

'You're very welcome,' I said. 'And good luck.'

I really hadn't done very much, but I'd learned over the years that sometimes just being a trusty shoulder to cry on can be a tremendous help.

The following year, in 2002, my niece Tijen announced she was getting married to her boyfriend Piet. She had been so strong since Kerem's death, and it was wonderful to have a happy event in the family. The wedding was in Göcek in Turkey and the ceremony took place on a galleon in the Mediterranean. Sadly, I was not able to attend as I stayed home to look after my dad, to enable my mum to go. The wedding photos were lovely, though, and I was so delighted for Tijen. Life was moving on for all the family, just as it should.

At Christmas, Peter and I had the great excitement of having beautiful little Tara to visit. She was at that magical age of eighteen months old, and completely stole the show. Elida was doing well, coping as a single parent despite her enormous loss. Seeing Tara opening presents and toddling around my sitting room was extremely uplifting. Though I hadn't seen her for a long time by now, I found myself thinking of ladies like Kimberley who desperately wanted a child, and I focused on the wonderful gift of Tara.

I think Peter read my mind.

'She's a little ray of sunshine, isn't she?' he said when everybody had gone to bed.

'She certainly is,' I said. 'We're all very lucky to have her.'

Unbelievably, just a few days later I was out shopping in Glossop when I heard an excited voice calling out: 'Linda! Linda!'

I turned around to see Kimberley walking towards me, across the shoppers' car park.

'Guess what? I'm pregnant!' she said.

It must have been twelve months since I'd last seen her, and it completely took my breath away.

'That's *wonderful* news! I was literally just thinking about you the other day. I must be psychic! How many weeks are you?'

'Fourteen,' she beamed.

We both knew that getting past the first twelve weeks is very important for someone with a history of miscarriage, and I wished her the very best of luck.

'I might see you at the antenatal clinic. I hope so.'

It was 2 January 2003, and a quick mental calculation told me her baby would be due around June. I would make a point of looking out for her name at the clinic.

Six weeks later, at her 20-week check, I did indeed see Kimberley at antenatal clinic, but I was concerned to see that she looked very anxious and worried, even though her pregnancy was progressing well. I completely understood how she felt, having waited so long for this baby, and I gave her extra support.

She introduced me to her mum and her husband, and I felt I knew her extremely well by the end of her pregnancy. Her bump was never very big, which worried her no end, and I was forever pointing out that she was a petite woman, and that having a small bump was normal.

Her daughter Beth was born at the end of May, a few weeks early and weighing five pounds, nine ounces. I didn't actually deliver her, as I was on holiday at the time, but I heard from my colleague that the delivery was perfectly normal, and the baby was absolutely fine. Kimberley, of course, was thrilled beyond measure. I was absolutely delighted, too, and I couldn't wait to visit.

'Is it OK to pop round?' I asked Kimberley's husband when he answered the phone.

'Of course. Kimberley has a little gift for you. It will be lovely to see you.'

Beth was an extremely pretty little baby, and her mum had a permanent smile on her face the whole time I was there.

'Thank you, Linda,' she said, handing me a little figure of a guardian angel. 'This is for you. That is what you have been to me.'

Chapter Sixteen

'Now we have four midwives!'

In January 2005 I was dispatched to an address in the centre of Ashton, where a Polish lady called Halina had gone into labour. She was not due until the following week and had not planned to have a home birth, but from what my colleague who took the call on the labour ward could gather, things were happening quickly and so an ambulance had also been sent to her home. 'Her husband didn't speak great English but it sounded urgent,' my colleague said. 'He told me: "She need help now. Right now. Please send ambulance. Baby is coming" and then hung up.'

I had actually been on my way into the hospital to pick up some notes for another patient who was expecting me to call in for a home visit, and so I quickly postponed that appointment and dashed to the address just off Warrington Street. The ambulance pulled up at the same time as I did, and I laughed when I saw that my old colleague Barry was one of the ambulancemen on duty. He was now silver-haired and he'd been ribbing me for thirty-odd years about that time one of our ladies gave birth in a washing-up bowl in the toilet, while I finished my cuppa.

'I'll not say a word,' he chortled this time. 'Except to say you'll be glad to know I'm retiring this year, so I'll finally have to stop pulling your leg, Linda!'

'You know I don't mind,' I smiled. 'And I wish you all the best for your retirement.'

A very earnest-looking young man threw open the front door and implored us to come inside quickly. 'Halina is having baby very soon. Please be fast. I am Aleksy.'

Barry said he would wait in the hallway while I stepped into the lounge of the small, semi-detached house. I was taken aback by what I saw. There were at least ten relatives of all ages crammed into the room. Halina was panting dramatically on the settee under the front window and there were three female relatives surrounding her, all with furrowed brows. They shuffled out of my way as I approached the patient.

'Thank you,' I smiled. 'You can leave Halina with me now. She is in safe hands.' The women nodded and retreated to the kitchen, herding the other relatives, including men and children, out with them. Only Aleksy stayed in the room, hovering anxiously beside the settee but averting his eyes towards the window as he interpreted what I said to Halina, who I quickly realised did not speak a word of English.

'Please explain that I need to examine her,' I said to Aleksy, who relayed this to Halina very efficiently. He continued to do a marvellous job of translating as I asked for specific details about when the contractions started, and how frequently the pains were coming.

'There is time to go to the hospital,' I explained to Halina. 'We need to get you into the ambulance. Do you think you can manage to walk?'

Halina nodded as soon as she understood, and I got Barry to help me escort her into the ambulance while Aleksy went to relay what was happening to the other relatives, one of whom decided to follow us in his car.

'Come on, Aleksy,' I called through to the kitchen. 'Let's go!' I directed him swiftly into the ambulance, and we travelled to the maternity unit with the blue light flashing and Halina moaning with pain but managing well in the circumstances. Aleksy, by contrast, looked incredibly uncomfortable and I suggested that he might want to hold his wife's hand. This wouldn't reduce her pain, of course, but I found it usually helped calm the atmosphere if the husband had a job to do, instead of sitting awkwardly on the sidelines, and I felt Aleksy needed to relax a bit.

'She is not my wife,' he blurted, as I signalled to him to take hold of Halina's hand. 'I am the family translator. Her husband is following in his car.'

'Oh, I see,' I said, hopefully without revealing that my heart had skipped a beat in surprise. 'Well, thank you for coming with us. It is very kind of you indeed.'

Halina didn't seem to care one bit, which was a relief, and though it crossed my mind to explain that I wouldn't normally invite a man who was not the patient's husband or close relative into the ambulance, I decided not to bother explaining the mix-up to her.

'Oh good, we're here already,' I remarked as we pulled into the hospital grounds. 'That's good. Very good indeed.'

I did not deliver Halina's baby myself, as there was enough time to book her into the labour ward in the normal way, but I did make a point of explaining exactly who was who to my colleague so nobody else made the same mistake I did! The next day I found out Halina had had a healthy little boy and was doing very well indeed. Her husband was with her for the birth and Aleksy hovered outside in the corridor in case he was needed, which thankfully he wasn't, as the delivery went very smoothly.

It wasn't until a few days later that I really thought about Barry's announcement that he was retiring, and I was quite taken aback by my reaction. I couldn't believe that this old colleague would be leaving, although it really should not have come as any surprise at all, as I knew roughly how old Barry was. What really struck me, I suppose, was that he and I were peers, and that my retirement was not too far off, either. This had been in the back of my mind for a few years, of course, but seeing Barry had made my own retirement feel that little bit closer.

I discussed it with Helen one day, telling her I wanted to work for as long as possible, and that I would stay on right through until March 2008, when I turned sixty.

'Well then, I'd better have my next baby soon,' she joked.

'Don't rush on my behalf,' I laughed. 'There's plenty of time yet.' I think I was saying those words to myself as much as to Helen, as I really didn't want my days of delivering babies to end any time soon.

It was the following year, in 2006, when Helen actually did announce she was pregnant with her second child.

'Linda …?' she asked with a twinkle in her eye. I knew what was coming before she said it. 'Will you deliver me again?'

'Oh my word, I thought I'd done my bit already,' I teased. 'But, seeing as it's you, I suppose so!'

Her baby was due in April 2007, and this time round she wanted a home birth. This put me under a bit of extra pressure, not having the immediate back-up of colleagues at the hospital if need be, but I didn't mind. Helen and her husband Dean were very close friends of mine by now, and I wanted to help them in any way I could.

I don't normally get involved in predicting the sex of a baby, but for some reason, with Helen, I was absolutely convinced she was expecting a girl.

'No,' Dean said, shaking his head. 'You can't be right, Linda. I don't think I do pink very well.'

Dean is a big, tall rugby player, and I had to admit that having a son suited him really well. Little William was five years old now, and Dean enjoyed the rough of tumble of parenting a boy. I really couldn't see him with a daughter, but every time I saw Helen I couldn't help thinking she was having a girl.

On the morning of 20 April, I learned that my instincts had been right all along, when Helen delivered a beautiful daughter she named Anna. She did really well through her second labour, and the birth itself went very smoothly, with Helen remaining calm and focused throughout. When the baby actually arrived, she and Dean were both absolutely thrilled, and their joy at little Anna's safe arrival completely filled the house.

I don't recall any banter about Dean being the father of a little girl after all, or about my prediction coming true, as we were all so overwhelmed by this beautiful little addition to the family. Anna was simply gorgeous, and my heart was full of joy when I waved goodbye to the family at 5 a.m., promising to return later that morning when they'd had chance to rest.

I will never forget walking back into their lounge at 11 a.m. that morning. Dean was sitting on the settee holding his newborn daughter, who was dressed from head to toe in pink.

They were surrounded by pink teddy bears, pink balloons, pink bibs and pink cards and wrapping paper.

'You know, Dean, I think you do pink very well,' I told him, and we all cracked up laughing.

I was extremely proud to become Anna's godmother later that year. I have been asked so many times to be a godmother to babies I have delivered, but I have politely declined many times, too. I think it's a big commitment to be a godmother, and it's not a role I take on lightly. If I had too many godchildren I wouldn't be able to do the job properly, and so I have only four in total. Anna, of course, was a very welcome addition to that little list.

When I actually did celebrate my sixtieth birthday in March 2008, I had been planning my retirement for some time and thought I was finally ready for it. I had been working in the NHS for forty-two years all told, and as a midwife for more than thirty-eight of those years. It was high time to put my delivery pack down and put my feet up. That's what I told myself.

I'd been paying superannuation for many years, and would qualify for a respectable pension. Colleagues told me how lucky I was to have reached retirement age. I was very happily married to Peter and we could spend even more time together. I could also see more of Jonathan and Fiona, who had both stayed local once they left home and settled in jobs. Jonathan was teaching 3D design at Loreto College in Manchester and really enjoyed his work. I think, like me, he had found his true vocation. Fiona was now a qualified accountant working as a chartered tax advisor with a firm in Stockport, and busily planning her wedding for 2010 with her boyfriend Pete.

As my retirement day drew closer, however, something didn't feel quite right. 'I'm really not sure I'm ready for this,' I confided to Peter one night as we sat drinking tea in our sunny conservatory, looking out at the fish pond in the back garden.

Peter had recently cleaned up the pond for the spring and, being an electrician, had fitted lights around it and added an electric pump to keep it clean. He absolutely loved tinkering around with such things, and I enjoyed the benefits of his DIY and gardening talents, which ensured the house was always running like clockwork and the garden was very well cared for.

I've always kept a tidy house, and Peter and I were a very good match in that respect. I think my strict nurses' training had a lot to do with my attitude to housework. I like things clean and pin-neat, just as my former matrons taught me. I was lucky Peter was of the same mind.

'What aren't you ready for?"

'Retirement. I'm a bit worried how I'll cope.'

'What are you worried about?'

'I think I'll miss my job.'

'Of course you will! You've worked at Tameside since you were twenty-one years old! You deserve a rest, though, Linda. You've worked so hard all your life. It'll take a bit of adjusting, but you'll be fine.'

Peter's words made sense. I was working full-time at this point, which was more hours than I really wanted, but there was no such thing as a part-time community midwife at Tameside, and I didn't want to go back into the hospital and work shifts. Three months earlier I'd actually asked Lesley Tones, who was now Head of Midwifery, if there was any possibility of cutting back my hours, but I was turned down, as such a post did not exist. It was all or nothing, and after speaking to Peter I agreed that I should not be working full-time in my sixties, and that taking my pension was the right thing to do.

Still, as I sat and thought that day, I felt quite unsettled. I liked the routine of work. I enjoyed the social side of my job, too, meeting new people and having colleagues around me. Most of all, I loved being part of the miracle of birth. Feeling a newborn baby in my hands still completely thrilled me, even after delivering more than two thousand babies in my career. What on earth would I do without all that?

My life at home was so neatly organised that I didn't have a stack of jobs on my 'to-do' list for when I retired. Peter himself was retired now, though he still did the odd small job for friends and family, which suited him well. I'd always been fortunate enough to go on holidays, both abroad and in this country. Whenever my brother John moved to another foreign country, I always visited. Having retired himself some years earlier, he now ran a wine bar in Turkey with Nevim, and I'd enjoyed several relaxing breaks there, soaking up the sunshine.

I also saw friends regularly, and my old school pals Sue Smith, Susan Thornley, Angela Faulkner and I still went out for meals together, just as we always had. The topics of conversation had changed over the years, of course. Instead of comparing fashions and talking about the hit parade, as we did in the Seventies, or worrying about our teenagers or the fact our hair was going grey, as we did in the Eighties or Nineties, we now discussed our children's marriages and traded thoughts about becoming grandparents. We also shared tales about our various jobs and pastimes, of course, and when I thought about 'the girls' I realised I didn't want to *stop* talking about my work with them.

I never dined out on stories about the ladies I delivered and was always very careful about patient confidentiality, but the arrival of babies is a topic women never tire of discussing, and I could not imagine a day when I didn't have yet another new tale to tell. Still, the wheels were set in motion now, and I listened to Peter and decided that he was still probably right. I would be fine once I'd got used to the adjustment. I would just have to make the best of it.

When my official retirement day arrived on 31 March 2008 my colleagues made quite a fuss of me and I had a retirement party in the hospital. Everyone said such kind things it made me cry, although that is not surprising as I have always been a sentimental person. I received a lovely figurine of a mother and baby, some beautiful flowers and lots of cards with wonderful messages. I felt very special on that day, but when I drove home I had quite a strong feeling that this was not the end. I wondered if I was trying to protect myself, or else I would have been so terribly upset. Who knows? But somehow, I sensed I was not going to accept that my days of delivering babies were over.

I was right, thank goodness, and it didn't take long for me to go into reverse gear. I was a lady of leisure for just three weeks before I got my job back, in fact. Lesley Tones telephoned me when I was watering the plants at home one day and asked me to pop in and see her. She knew that what I really wanted was a part-time post, and to my absolute delight she offered me the chance to work two days a week in the community, for a trial period of three months.

'I have given this some thought and I do not want to lose a midwife of your experience,' she told me. 'I remembered your request to cut down your hours. What do you say?'

I was flattered and absolutely ecstatic. This was the perfect compromise for me, and I could not have been happier. It felt meant to be.

'Are you sure you've made the right decision?' Peter teased one cold and snowy morning in the winter of 2009. I'd been called out to a lady called Suzanne Brookes, who was in labour at home in Glossop and was snowed in.

It was 6.30 a.m. and I wasn't actually on duty until 8.30 a.m., but because I was the nearest available midwife, I'd agreed to help. I must admit I wasn't entirely thrilled about this. I was warm and cosy in my bed for another hour, so I thought, but I dutifully headed out in my Daihatsu Terios 4x4, which Peter kindly helped to dig out of our drive.

The snow was falling heavily as I approached the address, which was down a narrow lane leading off The Fairways in Glossop. I suddenly had a sense of *déjà vu* when I saw an ambulance with a flashing light at the top of the lane. It was just like that time several years earlier – was it 2002? – when I'd had to abandon my car and walk the last few hundred metres through the snow to deliver Sarah Heywood's baby. I'd arrived at her house looking like a snowman, I recalled, and I sensed history was about to repeat itself.

'Good heavens!' the ambulance driver exclaimed when I parked up behind him and went over to have a word. 'Now we have four midwives!'

'Four midwives?' I said, suddenly seeing red. 'Are you saying I've been called out of my bed in this weather when there are already three other midwives here?'

'Technically,' he said. 'But I'll explain.'

It turned out that the patient herself was a midwife, and so were her two friends, who lived nearby and had come round to help.

'Oh, right!' I said, calming down. 'That's different. For one horrible minute I thought three other community midwives had been sent here ahead of me.'

I crunched through the deep snow down the lane for several minutes before the patient's pretty little cottage finally came into view.

'Sorry I'm so wet,' I apologised when a relative opened the door.

'There's no need to apologise. Thank you for coming. Please, come in. Suzanne's upstairs.'

I left my Wellington boots and snow-drenched coat at the door and climbed the stairs. As I did so I could hear voices coming from the bathroom to the right of the landing, and when I stepped in the room, three anxious faces greeted me.

Suzanne was on the floor with her two friends kneeling beside her. They introduced themselves as Debbie and Marie, both hospital midwives. I noticed quite a lot of blood in and around the bath, suggesting the baby had been born, but there was no baby in the room.

'I delivered the baby half an hour ago,' Debbie quickly explained. 'Baby's fine, but the placenta's stuck.'

Syntocinon, which is now the preferred drug to Syntometrine, had been given, but the placenta remained attached to the wall of the uterus and Debbie had tried to release it by pulling gently on the cord.

'What do you advise, Linda?' Marie and Debbie both asked.

I offered reassurance to Suzanne, telling her not to be

anxious as she had three professionals attending her, and between us we would take good care of her.

'Thank you,' Suzanne said quietly as I assessed the situation. 'What do you think we should we do?'

'Let's wait a little,' I replied. 'We have time. Where is the baby?'

'With Adrian in the front bedroom,' Debbie said.

'Right, I'll go and check the baby and come right back.'

Very often at a home delivery, the baby soon gets cold because houses tend not to be as warm as hospital delivery rooms. I've often had to heat baby clothes in a tumble dryer, or ask the dad to put the clothes inside his shirt to warm them, because if a baby's temperature drops he or she can begin making a grunting noise, which is a sign that all is not well.

I was delighted to see that Suzanne's baby girl was lovely and warm and pink, wrapped in a blanket and tucked inside her daddy's jacket, no doubt on the advice of Debbie and Marie. I had no concerns about her at all, and so I went straight back to the bathroom.

Debbie and Marie both looked to me for guidance once more, and I could see that they were a little out of their comfort zone. All three women worked at Salford Royal and Suzanne had booked to have her baby there, before the snow changed her plans. They were all experienced hospital midwives, but *this* was my domain.

'What's the best thing to do, Linda?' Marie asked.

Suzanne was coping well in the circumstances. This was not an emergency situation yet, but I knew that if we didn't act quickly things could go terribly wrong, as the patient may start to haemorrhage. Looking at the amount of blood already in the bathroom, I decided Suzanne should go to hospital, despite the snow.

I think all three women were glad I'd made the decision, and I told them I'd have a quick word with the ambulance driver and ask if Suzanne could be taken to Salford instead of Tameside Hospital.

'We need some clothes and some big knickers,' I said to Adrian, who jumped into action at once while Marie held the baby and I spoke to one of the ambulance crew.

'Seeing as it's you,' the ambulanceman said kindly, and Suzanne was delighted she was being taken to Salford, where she would feel much more at home than in Tameside.

Within a few minutes we had everything organised. Debbie would go in the ambulance with Suzanne and she would be able to write up her notes on the way. Marie would follow with Adrian and the baby in the car.

I wrote up a few notes myself, but once this decision was taken I really wanted to move Suzanne as soon as possible. The crew had managed to get the ambulance nearer to the cottage, which was good, and within fifteen minutes of the decision being made to take her in, Suzanne was on her way. I felt relieved as I watched the ambulance drive away. I knew this was the correct decision, and that even if the journey was slow through the snow, Suzanne was certainly safer now than she was on her bathroom floor.

I visited Suzanne back at the cottage four days later. She had had to go to theatre for a manual removal of her placenta, but all was well afterwards and her daughter, Maisy, was thriving. We talked about her experience several times during my postnatal visits, and Suzanne was a lovely, caring person; someone I knew must be a good midwife. On my last visit she gave me a little gift and told me: 'If you are an example of Tameside midwives I will never hesitate to have my next baby there.' It was a lovely compliment, and one I treasured.

At the start of 2010 I received an invitation to help promote a new service offered across Greater Manchester called 'Direct to Midwife'. The initiative meant pregnant women could call a direct phone number to speak to a midwife as soon as they found out they were pregnant, and antenatal care could begin sooner than if they went through their GP.

I fully supported the initiative and, in the light of my experience with Halina, my Polish patient, I was particularly pleased to see that there would also be a translation service on offer to help women whose first language was not English. I was delighted, too, to discover that Julie Hesmondhalgh was backing the campaign, and that she had agreed to help publicise it by inviting a number of local midwives on to the set of *Coronation Street*.

It was now more than eight years since Martha Mo's birth and I didn't want to make a fuss about the fact I had been Julie's midwife through her pregnancy, but as soon as she spotted me standing on the cobbles outside the Rovers Return she came rushing over and beamed: 'Look everybody, this is Linda. This is *my* midwife!' She went on to say what excellent care she had received at Tameside, and thanked me for being so caring and supportive. We posed for a photograph together and I felt really proud of myself, and my profession.

I remember showing my daughter Fiona the subsequent newspaper article that appeared in the *Tameside Advertiser* on 18 February 2010.

'Mum, I'm so proud of you,' she told me. 'Will you be my midwife, when I get pregnant?'

'That goes without saying. Of course I will, but you'll probably drive me mad. I know what a little worrier you are!'

Fiona was thirty-one years old and was doing very well at her accountancy firm in Stockport. She and her husband Pete made a terrific couple, and their wonderful big white wedding on 18 September 2009 had been a day full of joy. I could not have been happier that my daughter was now thinking about starting a family.

'Can you imagine us being grandparents?' I said excitedly to Peter that evening, after relaying my conversation with Fiona to him. His only daughter Sharon had no children, and if everything went to plan for Fiona, her baby would be *our* very first grandchild.

'Oh, it'd be marvellous,' Peter replied. 'But are you sure you'd want to *deliver* your own grandchild?'

I didn't want to tempt fate by talking in too much detail about something that was only hypothetical at this stage, but I answered without hesitation.

'No, I don't think that would be right. I think it would be too much pressure for us both. I'd want to be Fiona's midwife through her pregnancy, but the delivery is a different matter.'

'That's good to hear,' Peter said. 'I think that's very wise. I wouldn't want you to have too much on your plate, Linda.'

I squeezed my husband's hand and felt a deep outpouring of love for him. Peter was a dear, kind man. He always had my best interests at heart and, throughout our years together, he had done nothing but put me first.

Very sadly, by the time Fiona announced she was pregnant a few months later, Peter had been diagnosed with cancer. He did not feel ill but had gone to the doctor as a precaution, after failing to shake off a cough he'd had for a month or so. The doctor sent him for a chest X-ray and, to our absolute shock and dismay, Peter was told he had lung cancer.

I really couldn't take the news in. I think I must have been slightly in denial, to be truthful, because even though the diagnosis was very clear and we were told the prognosis was not good, I didn't see Peter as an ill person at all. I certainly didn't treat him that way, either, because he didn't behave any differently. He was as thoughtful and supportive as he's always been, if not more so, and our life carried on, albeit with a cloud hanging over us.

'Now promise me you won't worry too much about Fiona?' he said many times in the early months of Fiona's pregnancy. 'I don't want *either* of you getting stressed. I want you to enjoy this time, looking forward to the baby coming.'

'Peter! I'm the one who should be looking after you! I'm fine, honestly I am. Now don't *you* start worrying about me.'

I was absolutely thrilled that Fiona was pregnant and it helped so much to focus on such positive news within the family, but I also felt a pang of sorrow whenever Peter talked about the baby and the future. The unpalatable truth was we didn't know what the future held for him, and yet here he was, thinking only of me and my well-being, and the health of my daughter.

Fiona's baby was due in August 2011. I explained my reservations about actually delivering her, and Fiona understood completely. She decided she would have the baby at Tameside, delivered by whichever midwife was on duty, and she was happy with that arrangement. I would be Fiona's midwife throughout her pregnancy and I would be with her at the birth, but I would not have the responsibility of delivering her.

We thought we had it all worked out, and I lost count of the number of people who remarked what a lucky girl Fiona was to have such an experienced midwife for a mum. It was almost as if my involvement would magically make Fiona's pregnancy and birth easier. Of course, my experience had taught me that you can never, ever predict how life's big moments will turn out.

Tragically, Peter did not live to see the baby. His death came very quickly, at the end of February 2011, when Fiona was just three months pregnant. His funeral was one of the saddest days of my life. He was such a very good man, and I missed everything about him. I think I experienced every emotion known to woman in the weeks and months surrounding his passing. He suffered for a short time at the end, and I was glad his pain was over. I was very grateful for the thirteen happy years we spent together, but I also felt so bereft and cross that he had gone so soon. He was only seventy-one years old.

Each day I tried to take a leaf out of Peter's book. He was a positive person, and I tried to concentrate on what I had, not what I had lost. I put a photograph of him into a silver frame and placed it on the mantelpiece of the fireplace in my sitting room, and I cherished the happy memories we had made together. He would not want me to sit at home and cry, and I made an effort each day to put a smile on my face, and to try to make other people smile, too.

'Mum, I've got terrible backache,' Fiona told me one night on the phone, in July 2011. She'd done a full day's work and had then been out in the evening to have a 3D baby scan, as her neighbour was a midwife at nearby Oldham Hospital and had asked Fiona if she would volunteer to demonstrate the new scanner to other women.

'You've probably just overdone it today,' I told Fiona. 'When you've been at work all day you need to just go home and put your feet up.'

She was nearly thirty-five weeks pregnant and I told her to have a relaxing bath and get herself into bed before 10 p.m. She agreed, but at 1 a.m. my phone rang again, waking me from a deep sleep.

'Mum, I'm still in pain. What shall I do?'

'Get Pete to take you to the hospital,' I said instinctively. 'I'll meet you there.'

I went into autopilot, dressing quickly and beating a well-driven path to the maternity unit. All the while I told myself to stay calm and behave in the way I would with any other call like this. Fiona would be fine. There was probably a perfectly reasonable explanation. Her pregnancy had been trouble-free so far, and she still had five weeks to go to her due date. We'd all be back in our beds soon, having been reassured that nothing was wrong.

I dashed into the maternity unit and found Fiona being examined by a colleague. Straightaway, I could tell by the look on both their faces it was not good news.

'My labour's started, Mum,' Fiona said through trembling lips.

My colleague confirmed that Fiona was about two to three centimetres dilated and would therefore be kept in and given a drug called Yutopar to try to stop her labour, as well as a steroid to help mature the baby's lungs, should he or she arrive early. Unfortunately, the Yutopar didn't work on Fiona and it was considered safer to allow her to continue in labour. She did extremely well, reaching six centimetres dilated with no pain relief, and progressing to nine centimetres after an injection of Pethidine. Then, inexplicably, everything slowed right down. Pete and I offered endless encouragement as Fiona's spirits began to drop, and after four hours it was decided to put her on a drip to get the contractions going again.

'Mum, I can't do this,' Fiona told me.

'You *can* do it,' I reassured her, even though my heart was aching for her. It wasn't meant to be like this. I had wanted Fiona's birth to be just perfect, and I felt very sorry she was going through this ordeal. 'It'll be fine,' I soothed. 'Just don't get upset. Things have started now and there's no going back. You need to stay calm and focus on getting this baby out safely.'

'But it's too early! Will it be all right?'

'Sweetheart, nature has a way of dealing with things. It's early, but I've known hundreds of babies born much, much earlier than this. I'm sure everything will be fine.'

Pete kept looking to me and taking the lead from what I did and said, whether it meant offering Fiona a back rub or more words of encouragement. He was great. When her pain intensified as the contractions kicked in again, Fiona began to cry. It was suggested she have an epidural to help her cope, which I agreed was a good idea. It was duly administered, and once her pain seemed to be more under control, Fiona became more settled.

Her contractions did become so powerful at one point that the dose of her drip had to be swiftly lowered, but once that was done she continued to have good, strong contractions. Unfortunately, after another couple of hours, Fiona had made no further progress. Her premature baby's head was not entering the pelvis as it should and this, in turn, was not helping her cervix completely dilate. There was a danger her baby might become distressed, and it was decided she would need to go to theatre for a Caesarean section.

Fiona looked at me with pleading eyes, and I was so afraid for her, but I agreed with the decision, and I had to accept I could not help my daughter at that moment. I had been in that situation so many times before with other patients, but this was so very different. This was my little girl, and I had to dig deep and stay strong, because she needed my reassurance more than ever.

'A Caesarean is the right thing to do, sweetheart, you will be fine and so will your baby. You have been so brave and tried so hard. I am very proud of you.'

Fiona now had to be prepared for surgery, and it was agreed that Pete would go into theatre with her. There were several midwives around her bed now, including an anaesthetist. They were explaining exactly what was going to happen from now on. I knew my little girl was in excellent hands, but I left the delivery room and went out to the car park, where I wept and wept.

'Please, please, God let them be safe,' I prayed.

It had not been long since Peter had died, and I knew some of my tears were for him, too. It was hard without him.

When I re-entered the labour ward, Fiona had already been taken to theatre with Pete by her side. The rule at the maternity unit is that only one person can go into theatre with the patient. 'Blow the rules,' I suddenly thought, and I gowned up and dashed straight to Fiona's side.

'It's a boy!' Fiona said as soon as she saw me. 'A fine little man.'

And there he was, my first grandchild, on the resuscitaire, being dried and checked over by a midwife. He was a little miracle, and it took my breath away to catch my first glimpse of him, all pink and bursting with life.

I touched Fiona's face, as it was the only part of her visible beneath the green sterile covers used in theatre. I knew that all was going to be fine now, and I began to smile. Pete was grinning, and we all started smiling at each other, breathing easily again for the first time in many hours.

Joel Peter Heyes weighed in at six pounds two ounces despite being five weeks early. How big he would have been had Fiona gone to full term in her pregnancy, goodness knows. As he was premature, Joel was taken to the special care baby unit for observation. All was well, and he was there for just over thirty-six hours before he was back with his mummy on the postnatal ward.

Fiona made an excellent recovery after her operation and was soon loving motherhood. She had a few problems with breastfeeding and went through a spell of thinking, 'I don't think I'm a good mum,' but really she has done extremely well and made me so very proud of her.

I honestly wasn't prepared for just how much I would love baby Joel. I'm completely blown away by the strength of my feelings for him. As I write this he is about to celebrate his first birthday, and he gets more adorable by the day. I simply can't get over how much I love the little man.

A few weeks after Joel's birth, I was called to see one of my superiors. She explained that it had been brought to her attention that *I* had been the person who turned down Fiona's drip when her contractions became too intense, and she wanted to check if this information was correct. I told her it was, indeed, because I was the nearest person to the drip when this action was required. Strictly speaking, of course, I should not have touched the equipment, as I was there as Fiona's birth partner, not her midwife. All this had come to light, incidentally, because each patient's notes are thoroughly examined whenever an emergency Caesarean has been performed.

Once I'd explained the situation in more detail, the matter was soon resolved, but afterwards I found myself considering how much times had changed. How on earth would today's more bureaucratic NHS have dealt with Mrs Sheridan being left alone to breastfeed another woman's baby, young Sally Black giving birth in her Evel Knievel motorcycle helmet, or Sangheeta delivering her baby in an admissions room with no midwife in attendance, I wonder?

A little vision of Mrs Tattersall came into my mind. I remembered the day she left me to deliver my very first baby, all by myself. I wasn't a qualified midwife. I was a wet-behind-the-ears pupil midwife, learning the ropes from my community midwife mentor. Had Mrs Tattersall followed the rules to the letter I would not have been left alone to deliver Lorinda Louise Willis back in September 1970. No doubt my wily mentor didn't make it clear on her paperwork that she slipped out of the house when the birth was imminent, but notes were never that detailed back then. She had left me to my own devices with very good reason: to give me my 'confidence case' as we called it, and it worked a treat. I could just see her now, lighting a cigarette with Mr and Mrs Willis as they sat around the cot and celebrated the baby girl's birth. There was no need for questions or explanations, because little Lorinda had arrived safe and sound. That was the most important thing.

'What's there to bicker about?' Mrs Tattersall would have said, had she been asked questions afterwards. 'Tell me that. I'm too ruddy busy thinking about the next birth to waste time worrying about the last one! Where's the sense in that when the baby's perfectly fine?'

Mrs Tattersall was always full of wise words. Joel was here safe and sound, just like Lorinda Louise and the thousands of other babies I'd seen enter the world. That really *is* what matters most. Regardless of the countless changes I have seen in the NHS and the mountains of red tape we have to deal with nowadays, babies just keep coming, same as they always have, and the same as they always will.

Epilogue

In December 2010 the maternity unit was due to celebrate its fortieth anniversary. One of my colleagues spotted an article about the milestone in the staff newspaper and began to laugh.

'Blimey, Linda, if you've been here since before this unit opened you must be one of the oldest midwives in the world!'

I burst out laughing. 'I'm not sure I like the sound of that. I might be past retirement age, but I'm not *that* old!'

My colleague decided it would be a bit of fun to contact the hospital press office and let them know they had 'the oldest midwife in the world' in their midst.

It was just a joke and I happily went along with it. 'I suppose it's quite fitting, really,' I told Peter one evening. 'I mean, I *was* on the original poster advertising the brand new maternity unit, so it'll probably make a nice little article.'

I dug out the old photograph of me, taken in 1971, which had ended up on billboards all over Ashton at the time, and later became the cover photograph of my first book *The Midwife's Here!* Peter had never seen the picture before and really enjoyed looking at it, and we spent quite a few evenings looking at other old photos and reminiscing about the past. I told him some of my favourite birth stories, and was amazed he hadn't heard half of them before.

'You know, this is really interesting. You should write some of them down,' he said.

I brushed this remark off. To me, delivering babies was second nature and was simply my job, albeit a very special job. I didn't think anybody else would really be that interested. It came as quite a surprise, therefore, when the hospital put a big photograph of me on the front page of their Winter 2011 newsletter and ran this story under the headline 'Fairley Special':

When Linda Farley started her first day at work at the start of the seventies the average house price in the UK was £5,000, a loaf of bread would have left families with change out of a 10 pence piece and the Prime Minister was just three years old.

It may be four decades on and a few things have definitely changed, but as one of Manchester's longest-serving midwives, Linda's experience and compassion hasn't altered as she continues to offer pregnant women in Tameside and Glossop the reassurance they need.

Soon after starting her nursing training in 1966 in central Manchester, Linda realised that her calling was to bring newborn babies safely into the world and chose instead to look into a career in midwifery. Her training started at Tameside Hospital on 1 January 1970 and after delivering thousands of babies she hasn't looked back.

On celebrating the landmark anniversary with colleagues Linda, who lives in Mottram in Longdendale, said: 'Working in a busy maternity unit is a team effort and although I have been sworn at, kicked, punched and even bitten on occasions, I still maintain I have one of the most rewarding jobs ever. Over the years I have become a professional friend to so many of the women I have cared for.'

Of all the fond experiences Linda can recall after delivering generations of Tamesiders, it is becoming 'the face' of the new Tameside maternity unit when it originally opened back in 1971 and the publicity photos she has kept that brings the memories rushing back.

Lesley Tones, Head of Midwifery and Women's Services at Tameside Hospital NHS Foundation Trust, said: 'I know that both the staff in Linda's team and the families who have benefited from her care value her presence and we hope she remains part of the team for as long as she remains happy to serve Tameside so professionally.'

I rather enjoyed what I thought had been my fifteen minutes of fame, and kept the newsletter in a drawer at home as a souvenir. However, that wasn't the end of it. To my surprise, the story found its way into the local and then the national press, which led to me being invited on regional television and the ITV breakfast show *Daybreak*, and subsequently being asked to write a book.

Peter was absolutely delighted for me, and offered enormous encouragement when nerves got the better of me and I didn't think I had it in me to become an author.

'You can do it!' he told me. 'It'll be a wonderful experience and you'll make a great job of it. What have you got to lose?'

Unfortunately, by this point in time Peter's health was very poor, and doctors had advised us that his cancer was not treatable and that in fact he may not have very much time left. I agreed to start writing.

My friends and family told me it would be a good distraction, a therapy even, and I really hoped Peter would live long enough to read my work. It seemed so very cruel that he might not make it, but in typical style Peter could see only the good in the situation. He refused to be maudlin about his health and instead focused on all the positives in my life, making me see opportunities instead of hurdles.

Around this time I also had the honour of receiving two awards. I learned I was to be given a Lifetime Achievement Award in the Cheshire Woman of the Year awards, and I was also nominated as a Community Midwife of the Year by the *British Journal of Midwifery*. Both award ceremonies would take place in spring 2011. I knew Peter would not be well enough to be at my side when I travelled to hotels in Chester and London to pick up the trophies, but I hoped he'd be well enough to hear all about the two exciting occasions. 'Don't you worry about me,' he said often. 'You deserve this recognition. Make sure you enjoy every minute.'

Sadly, Peter died before the award ceremonies, and just at the point when I began to write my first book. Right up until the end he told me: 'You can do it!' each time I doubted myself. 'It'll be fantastic, I know it will, Linda.' I am very sorry that Peter did not live long enough enjoy the success of *The Midwife's Here!* or to read this book. He'd have been more proud of me than ever, if that were possible, and I smile at his photograph every day, because I know he wanted me to be happy.

Of course, Peter also missed out on meeting Joel, which is such a shame. When I held my grandson in my arms he felt like the only baby in the world, just as my own children had when I first held them. This brand new little person, my own flesh and blood, reminded me very powerfully how precious life is. I'd always known it, of course. Each of the more than twenty-two hundred babies I had delivered over the years had reminded me of that fact. I would cherish life and look to the future, as Peter would have wished.

I love my family dearly, and they are what matters most to me. I am pleased to say that Jonathan is settled and happily living with his partner Katie. She also teaches at the Loreto College and they are buying a house together in Mottram. Fiona, Pete and Joel also live quite close to me, and I feel very blessed to have them all around me.

I appreciate my life so much. I have had my ups and downs, especially in my relationships, but my job has always kept me going. I can't describe how privileged I feel to have worked as a midwife for so many years. The women I have met along the way have taught *me* so much, helping to make me the person I am today. Thanks to them I feel wise and grateful and fulfilled. I am equipped to deal with whatever life throws at me, and to enjoy the journey.

That is why I want to end my book by saying thank you to all the women of Tameside I have had the great honour of delivering babies for. You are magic, each and every one of you.

Acknowledgements

It has been a life-affirming experience to write this book, just as it was with my first one, *The Midwife's Here!* I am very grateful to the many old friends and colleagues who have helped me recall the past. The memories have brought me a mixture of laughter and tears, each delivery recalled making me marvel at how very powerful nature is, what an absolute miracle it is to give birth, and what a great honour it is to be a midwife.

I would particularly like to thank the following people, who have all helped me to deliver this book, one way or another.

My son Jonathan, daughter Fiona and son-in-law Pete, who have always been there, telling me how proud they are that their mum is writing her story.

My brother John, himself a writer, telling me 'Yes, you can do it.'

My mum, who is now 93, and has always supported me.

My friend Chris Pearce, also a midwife, who, when I doubted my memory, said 'Yes, I was there and it really did happen like that!'

My colleagues at Tameside Hospital who have prompted my memory so many times.

The thousands of women of Tameside who have been in my care over the years, without whom my story could not be told.

Rachel Murphy, my ghostwriter, who is like one of my family now, and writes from inside my head.

Jonathan Conway, my literary agent, who would not take no for an answer.

Anna Valentine at HarperCollins, for having faith in me and for enjoying my first book so much she asked me to write this one. She and her team have been absolutely wonderful throughout.

Karen Sutti, who is the baby in my arms on the 1971 posters, and on the cover of my first book. Her mother contacted me recently to tell me that Karen lives in southern Spain and is married with two children of her own. I am sorry that I originally thought I was holding a little boy, but I held so many babies that day I could not remember which one became my little co-star!

Finally, I would like to remember Mrs Tattersall, my community midwife mentor who inspired me as a pupil midwife. She retired in 1981, and she passed away in 2008, at the age of 87. I will never forget her.

To enable me to share my memories accurately without treading on anybody's toes or breaching confidentiality, I have disguised the exact dates of some births and changed the names of some former colleagues and patients, but by no means all. I have of course tried to be as accurate as possible when recalling historical details about hospital life, although I would like to point out that trends at Tameside Hospital did not always correspond to national NHS trends.

**Read how it all began
in Linda Fairley's first book**

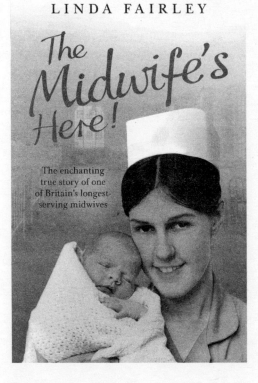

LINDA FAIRLEY

The
Midwife's
Here!

The enchanting
true story of one
of Britain's longest-
serving midwives

Prologue

'The midwife's here!' Mick Drew exclaimed, nudging his wife Geraldine as I approached her bedside.

Mick gave me a broad smile that was filled with a mixture of gratitude and relief. It was a look I was growing accustomed to seeing on the faces of husbands with expectant wives, and I had learned that the more imminent the birth, the more appreciative and thankful the smile became.

It was early 1971 and Geraldine was about two months away from giving birth, but she was in the highly unusual position of expecting naturally conceived triplets, which no doubt more than trebled her loving husband's concern.

'Flamin 'eck, how long? I'll go round the twist!' Geraldine had balked when I outlined her birth plan a few months earlier, explaining that her multiple pregnancy automatically meant she would be admitted to the antenatal ward in Ashton General Hospital for bed rest when she was seven months pregnant.

'That's the rule, I'm afraid,' I explained, thinking it was unfortunate Geraldine wouldn't benefit from our brand new maternity unit, which wasn't due to open until the end of the year. 'Don't you worry, we'll take good care of you in here and I'm sure you'll enjoy the break.'

Geraldine tittered. 'Well, I suppose rules is rules, though I'm not sure how my old man will take it!'

She and Mick already had three young children, and quite how he was going to cope alone with them while his wife was in hospital was not yet apparent.

'I suppose it'll be good training for him,' Geraldine said cheerfully the last time I saw her at antenatal clinic. 'Seeing as how we're going to end up with six! He'll have to get used to doing his share and keeping an eye on three of 'em.'

I was pleased to see Geraldine had an easy-going nature and was quick to see the funny side of life. She would doubtless need those qualities to cope with a brood that size.

'As for me, I'll just have to get meself a pile of good mags to keep me busy, won't I?' she winked. 'I'm sure I'll cope.'

It hadn't taken Geraldine long to settle herself into the ante-natal ward, aided amiably by Mick, who was a round, ruddy-cheeked man who visited often and had such a spring in his step he appeared to bounce down the corridor, flared brown trousers swishing round his ankles.

Every day he wheeled in a little tartan shopping trolley of provisions for his wife and greeted her by planting a huge kiss on both cheeks, and then on the lips. 'One for each baby,' he always beamed before handing Geraldine a packet of sweets or a paper bag containing drinks and magazines.

'How's she doing, Nurse?' he always asked me earnestly. 'Everything as it should be?'

'Yes, everything seems fine,' I reassured him. 'Your wife is doing very well indeed.'

'Terrific!' he grinned. 'She's a coper, my Geraldine, that she is.'

'In't he a smasher, Nurse?' Geraldine would often say after his visits. 'I've got meself a real diamond in Mick, that's for sure.'

I got so used to seeing Geraldine plumped up on a pillow, swathed in a garish purple satin nightgown Mick had bought her at Stockport market, that after just a few weeks it felt as if she'd always been with us. Sometimes she even talked the nurses into letting her help out with the tea trolley, dishing out cuppas to other patients.

'Does me good to stretch me legs,' she'd grin as she waddled round the ward shouting out, 'Two sugars as usual, Mrs Crowe? Best keep your strength up!'

'Evening, Nurse!' she'd always bellow when I turned up for a shift. 'How are you tonight?'

'It's me who should be asking you that,' I'd laugh, marvelling at how much energy Geraldine had in her condition. 'I'll be round later, make sure you're OK.'

When a woman is expecting triplets she is at greater risk of developing high blood pressure, protein in the urine and oedema of the ankles, all of which are complications that can threaten the safety of the mother and baby.

I knew Geraldine wasn't averse to sneaking to the toilets for a cigarette because I often smelled it on her breath, so I was always very particular about checking her blood pressure, in case smoking affected it.

Mick smuggled in the cigarettes, usually hidden in the paper bag he brought beneath a bottle of Vimto, a copy of *Woman's Weekly* and a quarter of pineapple cubes from the corner shop. He tried to be fairly discreet about the cigarettes, but Geraldine didn't really care if she got caught smoking, and often left empty packets and dog ends on the locker beside her bed.

One night as I sat beside Geraldine for a routine blood pressure check, I asked her how she was feeling being stuck in hospital for so long.

'Right as rain,' she chirped. 'To tell you the truth, you were right. I'm enjoying the rest.'

Lowering her voice and staring down at her wedding ring, she added bashfully: 'I'm glad I don't have to face 'im indoors all the time, too.'

'Whatever do you mean?' I asked. 'Mick thinks the world of you, and I thought you said he was a diamond?'

Geraldine leaned her head towards me conspiratorially and fixed her big green eyes on mine. They were glinting with what looked like a mixture of fear and excitement.

'Can you keep a secret, Nurse?' she whispered.

Before I had a chance to answer, Geraldine was mouthing the words: 'They're not his!' As she did so she pointed dramatically to her pregnant belly, which was now so huge it looked fit to burst at any moment.

My eyes felt as if they were bulging out of their sockets, but I tried my best to remain calm and composed in the face of such alarming and unexpected news.

'Well, I don't know what to say,' I blushed. I could feel the colour rising in my cheeks in preparation for her inevitable explanation and confession.

'You see, Nurse, I'm not proud of it, but I went out to a dance in Tarporley and got drunk. I was on those Cinzano and lemonades. Not used to 'em. I had a one-night stand and, trust my luck, I landed up with triplets! Can you believe it?'

She chuckled half-heartedly while I gaped open-mouthed and shook my head.

'No, nor could I, especially when I missed my next period and worked out the dates. Mick had been away, you see, got a big job laying Tarmac on the new motorway in Lancaster. You won't say anything, will ya, Nurse?'

I patted her hand and gave her a big smile. 'Course not,' I said. 'Why would I? Looks like he loves you to bits. I wouldn't dream of interfering. Now come on, get some sleep. Those babies could come any day now you're thirty-five weeks pregnant.'

I was absolutely stunned by Geraldine's revelation, and not altogether certain I'd done the right thing in playing down her infidelity. It wasn't my place to judge her, of course, but now I felt complicit in the deceit and I wished she'd never confided in me. That said, I found it impossible to be cross with Geraldine. She was such a likeable woman, as down to earth as they come. Her secret was safe with me.

The following night I arrived for duty on the labour ward to find an ashen-faced Mick pacing the corridor and dragging urgently on a cigarette, his brow deeply furrowed. For an awful moment I feared he'd found out the terrible truth, but he brightened immediately when he saw me and said: 'It's *very* good to see you, Nurse.'

It seemed Geraldine was in labour, several days earlier than anticipated.

'Look after her, won't you, Nurse?' Mick added, giving me a friendly wink. 'She's the love of my life, you know.'

His words brought a tear to my eye, but it was a happy tear. His sentiments put everything in perspective. He and Geraldine loved each other and they were stuck together like glue. Wasn't that what mattered most? I thought so, and I dearly hoped so.

As Geraldine had been in hospital for practically two months we were well prepared for the triplets' birth. The theatre was ready in case she needed a Caesarean section, but the consultant had decided to give her every opportunity to deliver the babies naturally, as that was the preferred option in the early Seventies, provided there were no complications. We had a team of staff briefed and raring to go, and there had been quite a buzz around the maternity unit for weeks now as we all looked forward to this moment.

I was very proud to have been chosen as one of the three midwives who would each deliver a triplet. It was unusual to have more than one midwife involved, but that was what the doctors had decided on this occasion. I was delighted to have a starring role in the proceedings, and I was also very pleased to have arrived for my shift in good time, while Geraldine was in the first stage, still labouring.

I quickly pinned on my cap, tied on a clean apron and gathered my notes before marching as briskly as my legs could carry me to the delivery room.

Geraldine spotted me the second I walked through the door. 'Glad you're here, Nurse!' she roared between hefty contractions that made her face contort beyond recognition.

Also gathered were two other duty midwives, Jill and Sheila, two trainee doctors I had never met before and two nurses I recognised from theatre and the neonatal unit.

I watched intently as the consultant, Dr Cooper, listened with an ear trumpet for three babies' heartbeats and announced to the room he was extremely pleased to report they all sounded strong and healthy.

My own heart rate was raised at the excitement of the occasion, but I wasn't nervous. Geraldine was a model patient – that's if you discount her frequent, ear-splitting cries of 'Bloody hell!' and 'Flamin' 'eck!'

She gestured for me to take her hand, and each time another contraction came she squeezed so hard I thought she'd cut off my circulation. We spent about two hours going through the same routine of screaming and hand squeezing and, as the labour increased, so too did the volume of Geraldine's cries and the strength of her already vice-like grip.

To help her cope with the pain she sucked on gas and air, which was attached to a big cylinder labelled 'Entonox'. We were ready to give her a shot of the painkiller Pethidine should she require more relief, but in the event her labour progressed so quickly and Geraldine was doing so well, there was no need. At about 11 p.m. the birth began in earnest, with the head of the first of the three babies visible, ready to be delivered.

'I can see baby's head. It's time to push,' I said.

'About bloody time. Aaaaarrrghhhh!' growled Geraldine, before pushing out baby number one beautifully, straight into my hands. It was an absolute joy to see she was a perfect little girl who was so fair she looked as bald as an egg.

As I set about cleaning the screaming baby, who was clearly in no need of resuscitation, I realised Dr Cooper had stepped in to deliver the second baby. He told us it was intent on coming out bottom-first, which wasn't what we'd wanted. Of course, having no scanning equipment in those days and only using our hands to palpate the abdomen and feel the position of the babies, it had been very difficult to gauge accurately how the triplets were lying.

I glanced at my colleague Jill, who had been meant to deliver baby number two. She looked disappointed, but we all knew that a doctor had to deal with a breech birth in these circumstances. Midwives are there to deliver babies under normal conditions, and this was a complication in an already unusual pregnancy.

Somewhere amid Geraldine's now blood-curdling screams and the hushed but firm instructions being issued by Dr Cooper, I heard the words: 'Well done. It's a boy!'

By now baby number three was obviously in a hurry to meet its siblings. 'Cephalic' I heard almost immediately, and breathed a sigh of relief. That meant this one was head first, thank goodness. 'And another girl! Congratulations, Mrs Drew!'

I looked at Geraldine's exhausted face and her eyes met mine. Often during a delivery the mother will seek out one individual for reassurance. Nowadays it is usually the husband, but with Mick still pacing the corridor outside, as expectant dads did back then, Geraldine looked to me in this room full of people.

'Well done,' I whispered. 'You've done it!'

It was only then she allowed a smile to stretch across her face. Despite her brave banter, she had been as apprehensive as the rest of us about this tricky delivery. So much might have gone wrong. Three babies meant three times the potential problems – and some.

'Are they all OK?' Geraldine puffed as I helped clean the babies up and arrange them in three cots around her bed.

'They sound it!' I laughed as the trio struck up a hearty chorus. They were captivating, they really were. Each one was perfect and pink and utterly gorgeous. 'And I can count thirty fingers and thirty toes,' I added, looking adoringly at each one in turn. 'They are wonderful! Shall I get Mick?'

'Yes please,' she nodded proudly.

I have never seen a man look as delighted and besotted as Mick did that day.

'Well, what d'ya reckon?' Geraldine asked as he stepped into the room, his dancing eyes not knowing which cot to peer into first.

'I'm as chuffed as mint balls!' he said, smothering Geraldine with kisses before going up to each cot in turn and cooing over his babies. 'Chuffed as mint balls!'

It was wonderful to witness a show of such pure, unadulterated joy and love. My heart went out to the Drews. They were now responsible for six children under the age of seven. Geraldine had already told me that Mick's wage only just supported them as a family of five, let alone eight. Now they would somehow have to find room for three more little mites in their small semi-detached house. With Geraldine not able to drive and certainly not able to afford a vehicle big enough for her family even if she wanted to, she would have to go everywhere on foot. She would be practically housebound, I realised, with a sudden pang of worry. How would they manage?

Looking at the Drews, who were now holding hands tenderly and gazing at their triplets through dewy eyes, you would never have guessed their world was anything less than perfect. The babies had been delivered safely and each one looked a picture of health. To them, nothing else mattered in that moment, and I was absolutely thrilled for them.

Geraldine and her babies spent ten more days with us. We placed three cots around her bed on the postnatal ward, and at night all three babies were taken to the nursery, where I would often feed one with a bottle while rocking the other two in their cots using my feet.

I felt sad when I finally said goodbye to Geraldine. Despite her smoking and cursing and despite what she had done behind her husband's back, she was a very nice woman who had a heart of gold, and I knew I would miss her. I still felt uneasy about the deceit, of course. I desperately wanted things to work out for the Drew family and I couldn't help worrying about what might happen if Mick ever discovered his wife's guilty secret.

'Daddy, baby Michael looks the spit of you!' one of the young Drew boys had exclaimed during an evening visit. 'Look at his big ears! He has your nose too!'

'What do you think, Nurse?' Mick said, directing a piercing gaze at me, which he held for longer than was comfortable.

'Don't ask me!' I laughed, sounding rather too jolly and wishing myself far away. 'All I know is you're a very lucky man, Mr Drew,' I added hastily as I busied myself writing up notes.

'I know, and my wife's a lucky girl,' he said, giving me one of his twinkling winks and smiling a wide, knowing smile. 'A *very* lucky girl indeed.'

He was a card all right, just like Geraldine. They made a good pair and I hoped they made it, I really did.

It wasn't until I was heading home after my shift that something dawned on me. Maybe Mick was trying to tell me something that night? I wondered if he knew the truth all along, or at least suspected it, yet he loved his wife so much he wasn't going to let it spoil a thing? He was a proud and staunch family man, perhaps so much so he was prepared to keep his wife's secret and raise another man's children. It was possible the only thing he wasn't comfortable with was allowing the midwife to think she knew more than he did himself about his personal life.

'A couple of cards all right,' I chuckled to myself when the pieces of the puzzle fell into place in my mind. 'Good luck to them.'